THE
MEDALLION
SOLUTION

39-0CON

THE MEDALLION SOLUTION

THE SICK HOME SYNDROME EPIDEMIC
OF THE 21ST CENTURY

DANIEL MOLLEKER

AND DANIEL O'CONNELL

To order additional copies of this book, contact:
Xlibris Corporation
1-888-7-XLIBRIS
www.Xlibris.com
Orders@Xlibris.com

CONTENTS

THE AUTHOR WISHES TO THANK THE FOLLOWING PEOPLE:

MANY THANKS TO DAN O'CONNELL, MY REMARKABLE RESEARCHER AND CO-AUTHOR, FOR HIS ASSISTANCE AND INVALUABLE HELP IN CREATING THIS BOOK. IT'S ALWAYS A PLEASURE WORKING WITH DAN. THROUGH THE YEARS, WE HAVE WORKED ON MANY SUCCESSFUL MARKETING AND ANALYSIS PROJECTS ALONG WITH INVALUABLE CONTRIBUTIONS AND CO-AUTHORING SEVERAL SUCCESSFUL BOOKS. A SPECIAL THANK YOU TO SCOTT SWIFT AND SCOTT MOLLEKER FOR THEIR INVALUABLE TECHNICAL SUPPORT.

EVEN MORE THANKS TO MY LONG SUFFERING WIFE, YVONNE, FOR HAVING THE PATIENCE, FORTITUDE, AND EVEN MORE PATIENCE TO DO ALL THE WORD PROCESSING, THE REWORKING, REVISING, SPELLING, AND GRAMMAR THAT RESULTS IN THE CREATION OF A GOOD BOOK.

WE MAKE A GOOD TEAM!

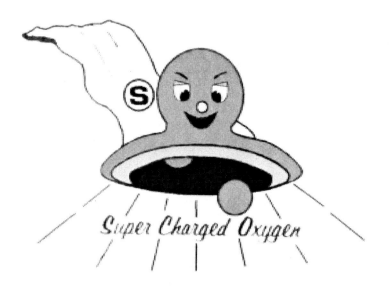

Super Charged Oxygen

SICK HOME SYNDROME

&

THE SICK BUILDING SYNDROME

Where did the words come from? Syndrome: (a group of signs and symptoms that collectively indicate a disease or disorder,—a running together, concurrence of symptoms.)

The Sick Home/Sick Building problem has existed from the time the human race began living together in some type of shelter. Although the words *sick home syndrome* may be relatively new, the problem is as old as the beginning of the human race.

Whether you live in a cave, hut, shack, shed, castle or house, there can be a problem involving the home you live in. Whether the causes are known or unknown, you have a sick home. It is a very harsh statement—Sick Home, consequently, the Sick Home syndrome.

Some people do not, cannot or will not identify with a *sick home*. Like so many things in our lives, *denial* serves their purpose until reality makes a shambles of their lives. "Other people have sick homes, I do not." "I keep a very clean home; it's impossible that my home is sick."

9

Most people would visualize a sick home as one that is littered with garbage, and very unclean conditions. In simple terms, that's where they are wrong.

In the first place, pollution and contamination, the bad things that are the primary cause of the sick home syndrome, are too minute (microscopic) in size to see with the naked eye. Just a few include fungi, spores from molds, viruses, bacteria, germs, microscopic insects, dust mites and their feces, pet dander, pet urine, vapors from degassing materials and products (carpets, drapes, furniture, rugs, cabinets, paint.) The list goes on and on.

The most common collection of symptoms reported by people includes; loss of energy, dizziness, headaches; dry, burning, itching eyes, nose and throat, watery eyes, and breathing difficulties.

Children and the elderly with respiratory sensitivity are most vulnerable. Allergies, depression, chronic illness, and asthma flare-ups have also been documented.

Some of the causes of the syndrome are attributed to loss of natural ventilation that contributes to the growth of fungi, molds, bacteria and viruses.

Treatment using environmental agents such as ionizers has been unsuccessful.

PREFACE

Recently, there have been numerous articles in local and national news media about sick homes; virus and bacteria influenced illnesses and the devastating problems as a result of mold, mildew and fungus. This problem has not only affected our homes, but also our schools, office buildings and in recent instances, our local, state and federal government buildings. People have been driven out of their homes, children out of their schools, and workers out of their work place. What is the problem?

In our rush to create more efficient and economically environmental habitats for ourselves, we have forgotten all about fresh air. We have effectively sealed ourselves in so-called efficient homes and workplaces. We insulate our homes with the highest R factor available for our area. We build buildings with windows that do not open. We rely on machines that attempt to circulate and purify the very air we breathe. High-rise office and commercial buildings, schools, hospitals, homes and cars, are all in tune with this ever increasing phenomenon of sealing ourselves in so that we can be environmentally correct with the dictates handed down in order to save energy. In the process, we have a generation of children growing up that do not really smell fresh air.

So, here we are, all sealed up and being very environmentally proper. What price do we pay? People are getting sick because we have forgotten all about real fresh air!

39-OCON

INTRODUCTION

How often have you or a member of your family suffered from some kind of discomfort generally assumed to be some kind of *allergy*? The truth of the matter is that the *allergy* may affect you in one way, perhaps only slightly irritating. However, another member of your family may be having far more serious and long-term detrimental damage as a result of the same irritant bothering you.

We know we live in a world of chemicals. In the process of constructing and remodeling our homes, numerous products and materials are utilized. These products and materials consist of many diverse combinations of chemicals and components. Everything from paint, carpets, drapes, floor, counter coverings and all of the other numerous components used in construction. All of these combinations of materials and chemicals constantly emit toxic vapors and manufacturing residue. This is known as *degassing*. This degassing is an on-going process for releasing the toxic vapors that help create an unbelievable chemical stew. Our homes may be energy efficient, which is shorthand for saying a humid zone of stale toxic air fueling a virtual soup of gases, all of which have some adverse effect on someone in some way.

Our concern in the development of this book is to illustrate how, through no fault of our own, we have been led into buying and living in homes, and other residential habitation that, due to the ill-informed myopic vision of

13

government, construction companies, engineers and building material manufacturers should, in fact, carry a Surgeon General's Warning on every door.

In the course of reading this book, it is our hope that our efforts will enlighten and inform you. We want to make sure that you and your loved ones do not suffer from the effects of the myopia of those who should know better. It is called the *SICK HOME SYNDROME*.

In the early 1990's there was an outcry of concern for the quality of the environment inside our homes, apartments, hotels, motels and workplace. Those who made the most noise have suddenly become quiet. Why? Their concerns were certainly on target. The energy conservation movement had spawned an entire new building craze in the 1980's. Houses, and every new living or workspace, were being sealed up and super insulated.

The unfortunate truth is that the media lost interest and went on to other subjects of more interest (in their opinion) than concern over the *sick building, sick home syndrome*. This syndrome can be compared to the Black Plague as far as incubation. It's sneaky yet approaching catastrophic proportions. However, the real tragedy of their non-attention is now coming home to haunt all of us. Worse yet, millions of people, young and old, are already suffering the consequences of all this so-called energy efficiency.

The incidents of allergies climbs, illness is rampant, more children are demonstrating asthma-like symptoms and other bronchial reactions. We now see TV commercials aimed at children who have asthma-like symptoms. While we sit in our energy efficient, super insulated homes, thinking we are all nice and snug, we are becoming sicker and sicker. We are exposed to more degassing chemicals in our homes than ever before. The EPA has identified at least 3,000 indoor pollutants! On the one hand, we have saved energy and perhaps some of us have lower energy bills. On the other hand, at what price?

That is what this book is all about; *CLEAN AIR.*

EXCERPTS FROM VARIOUS NEWSPAPERS AROUND THE COUNTRY

The Chicago Sun-Times—April 7, 2000 reports;

Local and federal officials are investigating a complaint that the Country Club Value Lodge Motel in Melrose Park may contain potentially hazardous levels of mold spore known as *stachybotrys*, which may be linked to respiratory ailments.

The Melrose Park Building Department plans to test air quality at the motel next week to determine if the spores—which have been contained to shuttered rooms—pose a hazard, town Building Commissioner Sonny Stamatakos said Thursday. The federal Occupational Safety and Health Administration is investigating a complaint by Merry Dailey, a motel employee who says she was sickened by the spores, said Angie Loftus, an OSHA official in Des Plaines. Motel representatives could not be reached to comment.

The Los Angeles Times—March 30,2000 reports;

Environmental tests planned at schools (Alecia Foster)
• Saugus district to check some classrooms during spring break.

Officials in the Saugus Union School District will conduct a series of environmental tests at several of its schools during spring recess. Seventeen classrooms at nine schools will be tested for things such a volatile organic compounds, formaldehyde, mold and carbon dioxide. The testing was recommended late last year by the state Department of Health Services after reports that classrooms were making some children in the district sick.

The Los Angeles Times—March 31, 2000 reports;

Judge Sues to Close Moldy Courthouse (Times Staff and Wire Reports)

A Superior Court judge is suing to close the Tulare County Courthouse in Visalia unless officials rid the structure of mold and fungi, which she says make her sick. Judge Elisabeth Krant alleged that a black, slimy mold contaminated the ceiling tiles in here chambers. The mold allegedly led to the judge's hair loss, dizziness, bouts of vertigo, abdominal pain, respiratory problems, ringing in her ears, facial swelling and severe rashes. Krant charged that county officials downplayed the extent of the contamination and concealed other information after tests were done in the courtroom. County officials have declined to comment on the lawsuit. In her 35-page lawsuit, filed Monday, the judge seeks unspecified damages in addition to a court order shutting down the courthouse unless the contaminants are removed.

The Los Angeles Times—March 31, 2000 reports;

Dangers at Home

MARINA DEL REY—Asthma is the most common serious chronic disease of childhood, affecting more that 200,000 children in the county, reported the Los Angeles County Department of Health Services, Public Health on Wednesday.

"The home environment may pose some very serious health risks for children and unfortunately, many families may not be aware of it." Said physician Jonathan Fielding, a public health officer for the county. "Moisture can cause paint failure and lead hazards, while mold and mildew are triggers for asthma and other diseases."

Characterized by coughing, chest tightness, shortness of breath and wheezing, asthma affects nearly 5 million children nationwide, and is the cause of roughly 3 million physician visits and 200,000 hospitalizations each year, officials said. Among infants and young children, asthma symptoms could include coughing, rapid or noisy breathing and chest congestion.

Musicians Register reports;

Hearth & Soul
The Fungus Among Us (Suzy Banks)

"Oh sure, discovering radium and polonium was pretty cool, but I'd rather have figured out how to get rid of mildew stains."

—Marie Curie after a couple of anisettes, as overheard at the 1903 Nobel Awards Banquet.

The Detroit Free Press—November 4, 1997 reports;

Mold has Proven Deadly (Raja Mishra)

The slimy black mold found in three Oakland County homes in the last month is a bona fide public health hazard that has

17

cropped up in more than 20 other states besides Michigan and caused numerous infant deaths.

The mold, *stachybotrys atra*, grows in areas that are constantly wet. Leaking roofs, leaky plumbing, sewer backups, and frequently overflowing washing machines can create environments for this mold. Studies show that when infants are exposed to both the mold and cigarette smoke, their lungs bleed and they can die.

"When we have a flood or sewer backup, we look for this mold . . . ever since the Cleveland cases," said Connie Morebach, vice president of Sanit-Air, the Troy-based air testing company that found the metro Detroit cases.

A little more than a year ago, 30 children in Cleveland were exposed to the mold and cigarette smoke. Nine died. At the time, doctors had no idea what caused the deaths and an investigation ensued.

Dr. Dorr Dearborn, a pediatric pulmonary specialist at Rainbow Babies and Children Hospital near Cleveland cracked the case. He discovered the link between the mold, the smoke and the deaths. He realized that most of the homes with infant deaths were clustered in old wooden homes with poor upkeep on the east side of the city. Three months earlier, a massive rainstorm had flooded much of Cleveland, producing conditions that promote mold growth.

In the Detroit area, the mold has been found in three homes, one in West Bloomfield Township, one in Macomb Township, and in Farmington. None of the residents reported infants with bleeding lungs. Last spring, one case of mold-induced bleeding lungs was found in a Detroit infant and one case in the

Thumb, according to the state Department of Community Health. Neither resulted in death.

The Centers for Disease Control and Prevention has recorded about 80 cases of unexplained lung bleeding in 24 states in the last four years, including two other cases in Ohio and 10 cases in Chicago.

Unexplained lung bleeding is rare: It strikes only one in a million children. In Cleveland, the rate was one in a thousand, a startling figure that promoted the study.

Sanit-Air found the three Detroit-area cases after testing about 20 homes, not for the particular mold, but for a host of contaminants. It is estimated that about 5 percent of all homes have the *stachybotrys* mold at one time or another.

Bloody noses and the coughing up of blood usually accompany pulmonary hemosiderosis, the bleeding of the lungs. The symptoms may be deceptive. Dearborn said six of the ailing Cleveland children came in with simple nosebleeds and were dead a week later.

THE FACTS

Q: What does the Stachybotrys mold cause?
A: Bleeding of the lungs.
Q: What are the symptoms?
A: Coughing up blood and frequent nosebleeds in infants.
Q: What causes the bleeding?
A: The mold releases toxins that weaken blood vessels in the lungs of infants. The weak vessels are irritated by cigarette smoke.
Q: How do I know if the mold is in my house?
A: Look in wet areas for wet, black and slimy mold, resembling tar or black paint.

Q: How do I get rid of it?
A: Clean the area with a solution of one cup of bleach and one gallon of water.

(AUTHOR'S NOTE: Whoa, not so fast! There is a real fallacy here. Get rid of it with one cup of bleach (brand name CLOROX) in one gallon of water? That cup of bleach (8 ounces) contains 6% sodium hypochlorite. The remaining balance in the cup consists of inert ingredients such as water (or 4.8 ounces of water.) Add one gallon (128 ounces) of water to this cup and you now have a total of 132.8 ounces of just plain old water.

After the sodium hypochlorite has spent itself, the moisture left over ounces (132.8ounces) as residue is plain old water. This watery residue environment has the capability to nurture tens of billions of fungi spores, viruses and bacteria floating around. This method has sown the seeds of the source to recycle even a larger crop of nasty stuff.)

The Sharon Pennsylvania Herald Internet Edition reports;

Asthma—Welcome to Ask the Expert

• Household Mold

Q: There is a lot of mold in my house in every room, in the basement, in the corners of the walls . . . etc. I also have a 6-month-old baby, and I have asthma. I am wondering if this is a health risk? Please send me any information on the dangers of household mold! Thank you.

A: Your description of mold is somewhat disturbing. In the last 5 years, we have discovered that one of the "wet molds" that can be harbored in the home environment just as you described can cause a serious lung problem with bleeding in infants. We have known for a longer period that for some people with asthma, molds are an important allergen (or substance when inhaled can cause allergic reactions.) Some people with asthma have no problems with one or more molds and others do.

Have you ever had allergy testing? If not, it might be useful to have testing for molds. However, the priority should be to protect your baby. I would call your city or county health department and ask to have an environmental inspector come out to your house immediately and test the mold. I would also go to your hardware store and learn how to get rid of the mold. You might need to get a dehumidifier because the worst kind of mold thrives on humidity and cannot thrive in a dry environment. The particular mold about which I am concerned is called *stachybotris*.

The Asbury Park Press of New Jersey—March 7, 2000 reports;

BOUND BROOK: Mom of ailing 3-month old suspects mold (Terri Needham)

Health officials are trying to determine whether a hospitalized 3-month old girl was sickened by mold in her home.

Jada Chambers was admitted to St. Peter's University Hospital in New Brunswick on Sunday, said her mother, Amy Stass. The girl has a double ear infection and a respiratory infection, and has been hacking, sneezing and vomiting, Stass said.

"They (Chambers' doctors) said it possibly could be environmental," Stass said. "I really do think it's the mold."

Chambers has been sick for three weeks, Stass said. She was recently in Somerset Medical Center in Somerville before being released and later admitted to St. Peter's.

A blood culture taken yesterday should provide some information on what the girl has, Stass said. She said her daughter is hooked up to a device that monitors her heartbeat and respiration.

Jada Chambers was living with Stass in her Columbus apartment before moving in with her grandmother in the Eastgate Apartments on the traffic circle two weeks ago. Both buildings were flooded during Hurricane Floyd in September.

Building and health officials, as well as an expert on molds, inspected the grandmother's apartment and an adjacent apartment yesterday. Officials today will inspect the Columbus Place apartment building. Stass said a white-and-brown mold in the basement there is creeping up to the first floor. In her second-floor apartment, layers of mold-like material have gathered on top of toilet water and water in pots, she said.

Three inspectors from the state Department of Community Affairs are scheduled today to begin inspecting places where there have been complaints about mold. The inspections will likely start at Blair House on East Union Avenue, where residents have said they are concerned about mold.

Residents are worried and local merchants have lost business, Councilman Frank Bruno said. "There's an enormous amount of phone calls coming into the borough," he said.

The borough is also obtaining special equipment to search for *stachybotrys*, a dangerous, slimy, black mold.

The Boston Herald—February 25, 2000 reports;

$1.9M Grant for Asthma is Nothing to Wheeze At (Doug Hanchett)

Boston officials are hoping to quell the city's growing asthma problem with the help of a $1.9 million federal grant that will help clean up the dust-filled homes of 500 asthmatic children.

"What we're going to do with this money is make sure that kids . . . have a place where they can breathe freely so they don't have respiratory problems," said Mayor Thomas M. Menino, who announced the grant yesterday at the Dimock Community Health Center in Roxbury.

Roxbury has the city's highest asthma rate, followed by Dorchester and the South End. And the ailment is the number one cause of school absences in Boston, officials said.

While the cause of asthma is unknown, scientists have discovered that mold, dust, cockroaches and animal dander often trigger attacks.

Lien Bigger, a 23-year-old mother of two asthmatic boys, Xavier and Joshua, said educating parents about asthma is key. "For other parents that don't know anything (about asthma), this (program) will help them a lot."

The Bangor, Maine Daily News—April 5, 2000 reports;

Airborne fungus found in Lincolnville School (Tom Groening)

LINCOLNVILLE—School officials learned Monday that an airborne fungus that could pose a health threat to students, teachers and staff plagues the Lincolnville Central School.

The fungus was found during routine testing in anticipation of construction to expand the school, principal Paul Russo said Tuesday.

As a precaution, Russo has moved one first-grade class away from the area where air samples indicated high levels of the fungus. In addition to the high levels of *stachybotrys*, moderate levels of other fungi and bacterial organisms were detected.

Preliminary research has shown that exposure to the fungus could cause coughing, wheezing, runny nose, skin rash, diarrhea and possibly chronic fatigue.

In a notice to parents, Superintendent Sue LaPlante wrote that the discovery of the air quality problems "is another in a series of challenging events for our school and community. We will continue to work diligently to ensure the health and safety needs of our students and staff are met."

The LA Times—March 31, 2000 reports;

• California IN BRIEF / SAN DIEGO

Hospital Blamed for Lax Crisis Response (Staff and Wire Reports)

Scripps Memorial Hospital should have done more to protect seriously ill patients from exposure to a potentially lethal fungus that thrived during remodeling and was also probably blown in from the helicopter-landing site, a state report says. A cluster of patients at the La Jolla hospital tested positive for the common fungus, *aspergillus*, from Oct. 28 to Jan 28, a time during which the hospital was remodeling. Six of the patients died, but an autopsy was done on only one, who had severe *aspergillus bronchopneumonia* in both lungs. "Without an in-depth medical record review, it could not be determined if ASPERGILLOSIS was the primary or contributing cause of death for the five other deaths," the report said. The hospital "failed to prevent and control *aspergillus* cases during construction" and "failed to maintain a sanitary environment . . . [which] may have contributed to the increased incidence of *aspergillosis* cases," said the 19-page report, disclosed this week. State investigators found a heavy layer of white dust coating many of the intensive care units' surfaces, such as beds, emergency resuscitation equipment, windows, curtains and nurses stations. Hospital officials defended the facility and said no patients have reported having the fungus since the end of January.

Press Release—Atlanta—June, 1997 reports; (Associated Press)

• Auto Air Conditioners—Fungus Farms
You or Your Kids Sick Yet?

That refreshing blast from the car air conditioner may be loaded with invisible bits of irritating fungus that can transform an automobile into a sick building on wheels. Some allergy sufferers, fed up with the wheezing and sneezing have even traded in their cars—only to find they can't escape it. "I wouldn't think there's any make of car on the market that you can absolutely say, This car is immune," said Robert Simmons, a microbiologist at Georgia State University who spends his days studying spoors.

The fungi, the same ones that can cause sick building syndrome, grow from pollens and molds that are sucked into the air conditioner. They breed in the wet, warm and dark coils in a matter of days. "Sick building syndrome has to do with allergenic particles or gases in an enclosed building," said Simmons, who has studied indoor air quality for almost 12 years. "A car falls under that same category and it is even smaller."

Simmons took samples from the vents in 27 cars in Atlanta—where cool air is critical to survival in the punishing summer heat. He found seven species of fungi that can aggravate asthmatics and allergy suffers and, "can make the car smell like a jock's shorts," said Simmons, who presented his study to the American Society of Microbiology in May.

"We're all exposed to fungus every day," said Dr. Jordan Fink, an allergist at the Medical College of Wisconsin. "They are out there, but they can be more concentrated in an automobile." Fink said two of his patients returned their cars to the dealer because they couldn't take it anymore.

The problem has so irked Chris Piotrowski of Folsom, PA that he's resorted to wearing a surgical mask in the car. "It makes me cough and sneeze and takes my breath away," said Piotrowski, who has bought two cars in the past four years in an unsuccessful attempt to eliminate the problem. "You turn on the air conditioner and bam, it hits you right in the face. It's disgusting." Doctors have blamed Piotrowski's breathing trouble on his smoking, even though he quit 23 years ago. The 57 year old says he didn't start to feel sick until after he bought a new car in 1993. "I do believe it is because of this, I really do," said Piotrowski.

Every year before spring Ken Wallingford spends most of a day cleaning and vacuuming the air conditioner of his wife's car. "My wife is extremely allergic to pollens and certain kinds of molds," said Wallingford, an air researcher for the National Institute of Occupational Safety and Health in Cincinnati. "She would wheeze and cough and have difficulty breathing. The car seems to trigger the problem."

Automakers and parts manufacturers are researching disinfectants, deodorizers and new coating to combat the fungus problem, said Simon Oulouhojion, president of the Mobile Air Conditioning Society Worldwide, an east Greenville, PA group representing 1600 manufacturers.

A mechanic can clean the air conditioning system with chemicals. Simmon's suggested that drivers turn off the air conditioner and keep the blowers on for a few minutes before and after driving. That helps to dry out the system. "That will go a long way toward preventing the problem. Air fresheners only mask the problem and offer no solution."

"People aren't going to get sick and die if they get in their cars," Simmons said. "But if you've gone out and paid $25,000 or $30,000 for a car, you don't want it to smell like athletic socks when you get in it."

Las Vegas Review-Journal—March 14, 2000 reports;

• Dangerous Molds Proving Unhealthy and
Costly for Homeowners (Joan Whitely)

Amy Riches loved the Las Vegas home she shared with her husband, Bill. It was heart rendering when they had to move out in October 1999 because the house was making her sick.

From the window of a trailer rented by their home insurance company and parked in the front yard, Amy Riches watched masked and suited workers empty the house of its contaminated contents, all ear-marked for disposal. Then she watched as more workers gutted the house to its wooden beams and studs, as part of the effort to rebuild it hazard-free.

"We are only allowed to take the clothes on our backs. (They told us), "Don't take so much as a paper cup. Don't take your makeup," says Riches, her eyes turning wet at the memory.

The villain the Richeses and their work crews are trying to eliminate? Dangerous molds; which the couple—and Dr. James Craner, a physician who specialized in environmental illnesses—believe caused Amy Riches' illness.

Sitting in a humble fifth-wheel trailer that is "the size of my foyer" in the house now under reconstruction, Riches runs down a list of her symptoms: unexplained nosebleeds, bloody coughing, balance problems, skin lesions, extreme fatigue, chronic diarrhea and decreased mental sharpness. The symptoms continue, despite medical treatment.

The mold was "black green. It was everywhere," is how Riches describes her first glimpse of strange growths found in the home in July 1999, when, on a whim, she peeled back some of her kitchen wallpaper to assess a decorating idea. "It was all over the back of it and on the wall. I sprayed it with bleach and called my insurance agent."

According to a report from Environmental Health Services, a local company that did testing for airborne, fungal spores, the Riches' 3,100 square-foot home near Blue Diamond had become an incubator for two molds, *aspergillus* and *pennicillium*, which are known to cause illness in humans. Not all molds that grow in homes are dangerous.

Water damage is the culprit, says the Richeses. It started with a November 1998 storm that damaged the roof of the house, which was built in 1979.

Water damage also is thought to be a culprit in the case of Terrell and Candra Evans of Las Vegas. In November 1995, they bought their first home, an older resale, near Rancho Drive and Washington Avenue. In September 1997, they bailed out after suffering various illnesses including asthma for their children and chronic bronchitis for the adults.

At a cost of about $2,000, the air was tested in the Evans' home, revealing the presence of *stachybotrys*, a mold that also has been linked to severe illness and several deaths in Cleveland in 1994. All the Cleveland cases involved children living in older homes with unrepaired water damage.

Stachybotrys also was found in the Sawyer Building, a state office at 555 E Washington Avenue, which opened in 1994. Numerous employees suffered health problems until the building was remediated. Craner and Linda Stetzenbach have written about the Sawyer contamination in a scientific book, Bioaerosols, Fungi and Mycotoxins. Stetzenbach is director of microbiology at the University of Nevada, Las Vegas.

When Craner visited the Evans' former home, "Right off, he thought it was musty, I think we got acclimated to it," Candra Evans recalls. A musty scent can signal mold growth.

Today, the house is padlocked and bears a bright red sticker from the city of Las Vegas reading: "Do not occupy. This building is substandard."

The Evanses have sued the prior owner and several real estate professionals for "insufficient disclosures to them" at the time they bought the house, according to their lawyer, Michael Duffy. Meanwhile, the family is living with Candra Evans's father and struggling to take care of the children's constant medical bills on a modest paycheck.

Duffy is a Chicago-based trial attorney who specializes in what he calls "toxic mold litigation." He also represents Melinda Ballard and Ron Allison, a wealthy Texas couple whose legal tangle involving *stachybotrys* in their 22-room mansion has been publicized by "48 Hours" and USA Weekend.

Duffy's livelihood depends on bringing landlords and construction, insurance and real estate companies to account for what he calls foreseeable problems that lead to mold-induced sickness.

"Pipes leak, roofs leak, windows leak," Duffy warns. And modern cellulose-based building materials such as Sheetrock drywall, acoustical ceiling tile and artificial stucco are ideal, when wet, from growing *stachybotrys* and other molds, he adds. "They will foster the growth of microbiological organisms, which will off-gas toxins as part of their life process."

Craner says he has treated about 350 Las Vegans suffering from mold-related health problems, as well as an equal number from out of state.

He doesn't agree with the language lawyers may use. "I call this indoor fungal contamination. That's not as sexy as 'toxic mold.' I think the (latter) term is a field day for attorneys."

Exposure to molds such as *stachybotrys* is rarely lethal, Craner points out. He says the media and legal hype has caused hysteria in some quarters, leading individuals to spend unnecessarily for expensive home testing.

And yet, the health effects can still be severe, Craner says. A leading stachybotrys researcher, Dr. Eckardt Johanning in New York, has told Ron Allison, the Texan featured on national TV, that he might have suffered brain damage from his exposure. Allison used to be a successful investment banker, but resigned because his mental powers of memory and concentration started failing.

"My expertise is . . . to diagnose and treat the medical disorder," says Craner, noting that symptoms of mold exposure can be mistaken for asthma, chronic cold or allergy problems. While the symptoms may appear similar, the mode of treatment should be modified. And the environment must be remediated, or problems will recur.

"The key thing medically, is many people are being mis-diagnosed," Craner explains. "Doctors are not even asking questions about their (patients') environments."

Like Duffy, Craner believes modern building materials and methods of construction make mold growth in new homes or commercial buildings more likely than in older ones. Besides the cellulose composition of today's building materials, centralized air-handling systems make the spread of spores easier.

When Candra Evans' family was forced to suddenly leave their home, she tried unsuccessfully to obtain temporary aid from charitable organizations that assist families who are displaced by disaster. She hopes they, too, will study up on mold; "When someone's in a fire, the Red Cross helps out. This is a tragedy where there's no help for you."

9-OCON

Las Vegas Review—Journal—March 23, 2000 reports;

• Mold Causes New Problems for UNLV Library (Natalie Patton)

UNLV's troubled Lied Library has suffered another setback with the discovery of dangerous molds growing in the unfinished building.

Workers this week are trying to get rid of moldy materials that otherwise would pose a threat to the students, librarians and books that this summer are expected to fill the $53 million facility.

The Public Works Board, which oversees work on state-funded construction projects, "has a remediation contract, and they're disposing of (the mold) right now," John Amend, the university's associate vice president for administration, said Wednesday.

Public Works Board Director Eric Raecke was not available for comment.

Amend and Kenneth Marks, dean for libraries at the University of Nevada, Las Vegas, said the university would not take ownership of the 301,000-square-foot building until the molds are cleared away.

Neither he nor Amend is sure of whether the environmental work will cause a delay in the building's opening.

Fungi were discovered and tested in early March.

UNLV microbiologist Linda Stetzenbach said two of the samples taken from four different areas showed the presence of *stachybotrys*, a mold that in some cases has been linked to severe illness.

"When fungi are growing on building materials in occupied areas, there is the potential for adverse health effects," she said.

Stetzenbach said an environmental contractor working on the unfinished library plans to bore holes into some of the Lied Library's walls to see if more molds are growing beneath surfaces. Building materials likely got wet during recent rains and flooding in July, she said.

The doors of the library, which benefited from a $15 million donation from the Lied Foundation, are expected to open this summer, at least six months behind schedule.

Problems with the library's construction have included the death of a construction worker, finding unexpected utility lines underground, stormy weather, floors that needed to be reinforced to support loaded bookshelves and inferior masonry.

U.S. News and World Report—May 8, 2000 reports;
Science & Ideas—Cover Story

• Allergy Epidemic

Everyone seems to be sneezing, and our lifestyle may be the culprit. But help is on the way (Nancy Shute)

The bright blossoms and tender green leaves of spring are supposed to signal a season of joy and renewal. But for millions of people, the tulips herald a season of misery: the wheezing and sneezing of allergies. Allergy, once the bane of a small, sniffling minority, is becoming epidemic. In the United States, up to 30 percent of adults and 40 percent of children now suffer from allergic rhinitis, the nasal congestion and itchy eyes commonly called hay fever. Indoor mites and mold plague many, and allergies to peanuts and latex are increasing.

Yet despite their ubiquity, allergies remain mysterious. Scientists still don't know why the human body mounts a scorched-earth defense against harmless substances and wounds itself in the process. It's unclear why some people can't be within hissing distance of a cat without breaking out in hives, while others are unfazed. Heredity plays a role, but genes can't explain the sharp increase over the past 30 years, particularly in developed countries. "Allergy's on the rise, and it's not clear why," says Ira Finegold, chief allergist at St. Luke's Roosevelt Hospital Center in New York.

Many culprits have been proposed, including pollution and changes in lifestyle. The most startling possibility: Allergy may be caused by the success of civilization. As modern life has become more hygienic, what with indoor plumbing, immunizations, and antibiotics, the human immune system has run out of things to do. It attacks allergens, and the body itself, as if it were bored.

Fortunately, for the first time in decades completely new allergy treatments are in the works. Using tools from molecular biology and genetics, researchers are devising once-a-month shots that eradicate symptoms, and vaccines that could make life virtually allergy free for millions. And many sufferers can get a large measure of relief from the treatments available today—if they're tailored right. Louisa Wirthlin, a 19-year-old sophomore at St. Louis University, wouldn't have dreamed of running outdoors in the spring until recently because of the risk of setting off allergy-induced asthma. Adding antihistamines to her asthma drugs has freed her to play soccer and jog without fear. "It's a very big difference," Wirthlin says.

Humans have long contended with allergies; hieroglyphics in the tomb of Egyptian King Menes record his death from an insect sting in 2461 B.C. Hay fever was first described in 1819 as a rare affliction of the privileged classes. As the country progressed, the allergy became troublesome enough for doctors to treat it in the general population. By the 1920's, clinics dispensing allergy shots had sprung up in New York City. Nowadays, the stuffy noses of rhinitis cost the United States about $4.5 billion a year in doctor visits and medications, plus 3.8 million missed work and school days and untold misery.

The problem is not just pollen but a host of seemingly unrelated triggers, including nuts, nickel, and latex. With people spending 90 percent of their time indoors, allergies to cats, molds and dust mites—microscopic creatures in the spider family that live in pillows and mattresses and feast on flakes of shed human skin—have become a serious health concern. Allergies to food and insect stings can be fatal, and allergies are the main trigger for asthma, which kills 5,000 people a year. It's no wonder that allergies have become big business for drug companies, as well as for chic shops and Internet sites hawking pillow covers and other allergy-control paraphernalia.

LIFESTYLE PROBLEM? Many researchers are convinced that almost half the people in the developed world are now allergic to something. Allergy consistently appears in the top 10 list of reasons for visits to doctor's offices. It's hard to document the incidence of allergy, partly because epidemiologists have tended to focus on asthma. But in some countries, including England, New Zealand, and Australia, statistics confirm a rise in allergies. In the United States, the numbers aren't firm, but reports of one symptom rhinitis, rose 31 percent from 1985 to 1995. The increases are too rapid to be caused by genetic changes. And people living in Eastern Russia, India,

Indonesia, and rural Africa report far less trouble with allergies, even though there's no lack of pollen, dust mites, and other triggers. "Something about the Western style of living has given rise to more allergies," says Doctor Leung, head of the pediatric allergy division at National Jewish Medical and Research Center in Denver.

At about the same time, however, epidemiologists noted that people who had serious bacterial infections in early childhood were less likely to develop allergy and asthma. Children born into large families were also less impaired. Erika von Mutius, the Munich pediatrician who discovered the Leipzig disparity, is now studying children who grow up on small farms in Bavaria, Switzerland, and Austria. These children, who often drink raw milk and live close to stables, have 75 percent fewer allergies than their village peers. "There seems to be something in a traditional lifestyle that's protective," von Mutius says.

Thus the "hygiene hypothesis": the theory that a squeaky-clean modern lifestyle somehow alters the immune system and predisposes people to allergy. But that's not the only notion in play. Other factors under investigation include changes in diet, exposure to diesel particulates, a decline in breast-feeding, less physical activity, and warmer, carpeted housing, as well as secondhand cigarette smoke—all of which might interact with the genes of susceptible people to produce allergy. "I don't think this is going to turn out to be due to one factor," says Scott Weiss, chief of environmental and respiratory epidemiology at Harvard University's Channing Laboratory, who is seeking genetic and lifestyle clues among villagers in central China, where people live much as Europeans did 150 years ago.

PIERCED NAVELS. Indeed, humans seem to have a perverse talent not only for altering the environment but also for introducing themselves to new allergens. For the first half of the

20th century, horses were a major allergy trigger. Now cars are more common than horses, most adults work in climate-controlled offices, and children play indoors after school instead of riding bikes around the neighborhood. As a result, indoor allergens have become a plague. Allergy to nickel has risen along with the popularity of pierced navels. And the increased use of rubber gloves in health care, a response to AIDS, has spawned a near epidemic in latex allergy, which has become a major occupational health risk in some fields.

Pam Purdy loved her job as a nurse in the neonatal intensive care unit at the University of Maryland Medical Center, coaxing premature babies through their first weeks of life. When the 36-year old resident of Forest Hill, MD started having trouble breathing back in 1995, she had never even heard of latex allergy. "The doctor knew right away what it was," she says. Purdy switched to latex-free gloves, but airborne particles from fellow workers' gloves worsened her symptoms. Steroids and other medications failed to halt her slide. "It was horrible," she says. "I thought I would never work again." She spent seven months doing office work before the hospital decided to make the neonatal intensive care unit off limits to latex.

In May 1996 she returned to the floor, apprehensive and closely monitored. She has had no major problems, but she can't stray from designated safe areas in the hospital and has had to convince her two children that they can live without toy balloons. "It's a daily, lifelong problem." The hospital now tests all new employees for latex allergy, and, like many other hospitals, is increasing the number of latex-free units.

Finding out what sets off a person's allergies isn't too hard. In one hour, an allergist can perform a skin-prick test, injecting tiny doses of allergens into the patient's back or forearm to see

37

which raise itchy red welts. Blood tests are sometimes used to detect antibodies to allergens such as latex. It's figuring out what to do next that's difficult. The allergist's first advice has traditionally been to avoid the allergen: Lose the cat. Banish stuffed animals and down comforters from the bedroom. Don't eat peanuts. Dust relentlessly. Stay indoors with the windows shut. Wise advice, perhaps, but hard to live by.

Allergy medications are also often hard to take. The primary weapon remains antihistamines, which were developed in the 1930's and block the production of histamine, the body chemical that causes hives, itching, and nasal congestion. But over-the-counter antihistamines like Benadryl and Chlo-Trimeton cross into the brain, causing drowsiness and slowed reactions. Nonsedating antihistamines, introduced in 1985, block histamine without the sleepiness. But they're prescription only, and expensive; a month's worth of Claritin or Allegra, the two most popular, can exceed $60. Many insurers balk at footing the bill, leaving patients with the unpleasant choice of being zonked out by the allergy or by the old antihistamine.

Many are choosing the over-the-counter drug, putting themselves and others at risk. Benadryl and other older antihistamines have been implicated in fatal traffic accidents, including several involving bus drivers. In March, researchers at the University of Iowa published in the Annals of Internal Medicine showing that drivers under the influence of Benadryl performed as if they were legally drunk. Other studies have found that people may not realize the drugs sedate them, even though tests prove they're impaired.

Allergy shots, in which small amounts of purified allergen protein are injected under the skin to induce tolerance, have been used since the early 1900's. They remain effective. But the shots sometimes set off dangerous allergic reactions, and the therapy requires frequent trips to the doctor for three to five years. Many people aren't willing to put up with the inconvenience, particularly for seasonal allergies.

Still, most people could be happy with the drugs now on the market—if only doctors prescribed them properly. For instance, antihistamines alone often don't relieve nasal congestion, but they do when used with prescription corticosteroid nose sprays such as Flonase and Nasonex. These sprays, used once a day, are "the gold standard for allergic rhinitis." Says Richard Lockey, director of the division of allergy and immunology at the University of South Florida College of Medicine. "They help almost everybody." Prescription antihistamine drops such as Naphcon-A or Patanol can relieve itchy, burning eyes.

Yet in a survey earlier this year, 25 percent of rhinitis sufferers said that prescription medication failed to relieve their symptoms, and 20 percent said their doctor didn't take their condition seriously. "Rhinitis is often viewed as a trivial nuisance disease," despite the fact that it can lead to ear and sinus infections or pneumonia, says Mark Dykewicz, an associate professor of internal medicine at St. Louis University who has worked on a nationwide task force to improve management of allergy. Managed care also plays a part. "Doctors are under a lot of pressure to treat patients quickly," Dykewicz says.

AWESOME POSSIBILITIES. Even people who most doctors would agree need help don't always get it. Wirthlin, the St. Louis University sophomore, had seen doctors since age 2 for her asthma. But even though she is allergic to pollen, molds, cats, and dogs, it wasn't until she changed doctors three years ago that the new allergist suggested she take oral antihistamines. She hasn't been in the emergency room in months and has cut way back on her use of corticosteroid inhalers, which can have bad side effects.

"Something like the right medication can change a lifestyle altogether." Says here mother, Shawn Tate.

The new medications in the pipeline may change lifestyles even more radically. "It's awesome," says Diane Miller, a Louisville, Colorado minister whose 12-year old daughter, Stacia, took part in a test of an experimental allergy drug. Before starting on the once-monthly injections last July, Stacia was so allergic that she couldn't play at a friend's if the house had cats or get near a horse without suffering hives and asthmatic wheezing. Then she tried an "anti-Ig-E" drug, a monoclonal antibody designed to hobble immunoglobulin E, and the human antibody that sets allergic reaction in motion. A day after the first shot, Stacia's nose stopped dripping and her breathing eased. Now cats are no problem and neither is horseback riding. "She doesn't have problems with anything," says her mother. "It's been great."

Researchers have sought to defang IgE since 1967, when Japanese and Swedish researchers first identified the antibody. They've known it comes into play long before most drugs. "The thought is if you can attack the disease very early, you may be able to treat it with a single drug," says Henry Milgrom, a senior staff physician at National Jewish Medical and Research Center in Denver, who conducted the anti-IgE trial that included Stacia Miller. That's just what the anti-IgE drug appears to do. Novartis Pharmaceuticals, the drug's manufacturer, plans to apply for Food and Drug Administration approval this year. Still, 15 percent of asthma patients aren't helped by anti-IgE—evidence that other factors besides IgE may be involved. Moreover, the drug promises to be considerably more expensive than nonsedating antihistamines.

As a result, researchers are looking for other ways to sabotage the allergic reaction. New tools of molecular biology make it possible to peer more closely into the complex chain of events and to craft molecules to intercept the bad actors. Anti-leukotriene drugs such as Accolate and Singulair, which combat inflammatory compounds produced by white blood cells, have proved useful for treating asthma since their introduction in 1996. They're now being tested on allergy patients, with promising results. Several laboratories are developing drugs to counter interleukin-4, which causes inflammation.

TEACHING THE BODY. New, safer vaccines are also in the works. Based on allergen DNA or on fragments of allergen protein, the vaccines would teach the body to tolerate the allergen without setting off life-threatening anaphylactic reactions. Clinical trials are underway on oral vaccines, which would deliver encapsulated allergens to the gut and avoid the need for shots. Buoyant researchers anticipate having new vaccines on the market within three years. And many scientists are working to track down the genes involved in allergy, the goal being to identify the people most at risk and tailor treatments to them. "It may be we'll identify children at high risk of developing food allergies and vaccinate them, just like we do with infectious diseases," says Hugh Sampson, director of the food allergy clinic at Mount Sinai School of Medicine in New York.

Even more appealing is the notion of not letting people become sensitized to allergens in the first place. The hygiene hypothesis—if it's right—could point the way. Early exposure to germs shapes a baby's immature immune system by bolstering the Th1 lymphocytes, the white blood cells that fight bacteria. Hygiene hypothesis proponents argue that if a child is protected from early infections, the immune system's other white-cell army—Th2 cells, which fight parasitic infections—will prevail. The Th2 cells also react to allergens, sparking IgE production and allergies.

41

Erika von Mutius, the Munich pediatrician who is investigating the allergic divide between farm and village children, thinks that microbes in the dust and dung of the stables may be prompting a protective Th1 response. "The farmers' kids are not sick," she says, noting that the children don't have more pneumonia or diarrhea as a result of the microbial cloud they inhabit. "They don't seem to pay a price."

The irony of suggesting that the cleanest lifestyle may not be the healthiest isn't lost on the researchers. But it may be that the human body just can't change as quickly as civilization. "We have lived with these bugs forever. That's what we're adapted to," says Fernando Martinez, director of respiratory sciences at the University of Arizona. "We super-ultra-clean ourselves in a manner that we've never done before."

Scientists are intensely interested in finding out how to push the immune system in the right direction. Yet von Mutius and other researchers cringe at the suggestion that public health benefits of the past 100 years should be jettisoned in order to avoid allergy. One study in Africa suggested that measles protects against allergy—yet 25 percent of the children under age 3 who contracted measles died of the disease. "We would do much more harm than good if we started scaring people out of immunizations," says Martinez.

PERPLEXING POSSIBILITIES. What's more, it's far from clear, which bugs would help more than hurt. One study published earlier this year in the *Journal of the American Medical Association* showed that measles isn't protective after all. Another recent report in the *British Medical Journal* suggested that the real immune benefit comes from intestinal pathogens. It might turn out that the key is the frequency of childhood diseases, not any particular infectious disease.

So molecular biologists are looking for ways to confer the benefits of dirty living without the risks. Researchers are already experimenting with "vaccines" made of *mycobacterium vaccae*, a soil pathogen that doesn't sicken humans, to see if it will encourage Th1 response. Others are investigating whether bits of DNA, called CpG motifs, which are unique to bacteria, can be used the same way—an approach that has already been used to reduce allergic asthma in laboratory mice.

But the ultimate goal in allergy treatment may be not to encourage one immune response over another, but to convince the body right from the outset that allergens are not worthy of an immune response at all. "The Ideal would be to be indifferent to these common and innocuous allergens," says Homer Boushey, chief of the division of allergy and immunology at the University of California-San Francisco. Boushey says it's something the human body already knows how to do; babies often generate high levels of IgE when they first eat foods like eggs and cheese. But over time, the infant immune system learns that eggs are just food, not an alien threat. Boushey is excited that laboratory researchers like himself are talking with epidemiologists like von Mutius. He predicts that these two arms of science will together decipher the enigma of allergy and usher in a future in which spring will promise nothing but delight.

43

PART ONE

CHAPTER 1

CREATING THE PROBLEM A BACKGROUND TO THE TOXIC HOME

WHY SHOULD YOU BE CONCERNED ABOUT THE QUALITY OF AIR THAT YOU BREATHE?

Most people are aware that outdoor air pollution can damage their health but may not know that indoor pollution can also have more significant effects. EPA studies of human exposure to air pollutants indicate that indoor air levels of many pollutants may be 2-5 times, and on occasion more that 100 times, higher than outdoor levels. These levels of indoor air pollutants are of particular concern because it is estimated that most people spend as much as 90% of their time indoors.

Over the past several decades, our exposure to indoor air pollutants is believed to have increased due to a variety of factors, including the construction of more tightly sealed buildings, reduced ventilation rates to save energy, the use of synthetic building materials and furnishings, and the use of chemically formulated personal care products, pesticides, and household cleaners.

In recent years, comparative risk studies performed by the EPA and its Science Advisory Board (SAB) have consistently ranked indoor air pollution among the top five environmental risks to public health. The EPA, in close cooperation with other Federal agencies and the private sector, is actively involved in a concerted effort to better understand indoor air pollution and to reduce people's exposure to air pollutants in *offices*, *homes*, and *schools* and other indoor environments where people live, work, and play.

Recently, there has been a legitimate and an undeniable concern for the quality of the environment inside our homes, apartments, hotels, motels and the workplace. This sudden interest was a direct result of the 1980's when building better insulated, less energy consuming living and working spaces was of top priority. Yes indeed, this was one of the many effects of the oil shortages and general energy conservation.

Across the nation new laws were passed. Insulation was the biggest winner as everyone scrambled to build homes with higher "R" factors. Millions were spent to re-insulate homes. The topic of conversation was how high an "R" factor you had or could achieve.

The path to the energy efficient house had its origin in the 1950's. However, energy efficiency was not the goal. Thermopane windows were introduced. The marketing ploy was that with double panes of glass and the air space between them providing better insulation, our homes would be warmer and there would be no more "sweating" windows in the wintertime. Without a doubt, the "picture window" was coming into style and, God forbid your window "sweated." Modern housing of the day simply could not be caught with a "sweating" picture window!

The Thermopane concept eventually made it to all the other windows in the house. Their use was a mark of economic status for those who had them installed in either old or new homes. Builders installed them to project the image of quality in their work.

The popularity of these windows was not found everywhere. In California, Florida and the Gulf States they were not considered a necessity because windows did not "sweat" very much in these climates.

The second major push in homes of the late 50's and 60's was the development of new gas and electric Central Heating Systems. The coal furnace was literally forced out of the basement by municipalities everywhere. These monsters, especially those burning bituminous (soft coal) had the capability of shrouding entire towns in a yellow fog so dense even a streetlight two blocks away was barely visible. Therefore, natural gas and electric furnaces with thermostats became *THE* item because they would make homes warmer and cleaner.

The next influence to enter the home was finding a way to make summer more bearable. In the rural areas of the United States, trees and porches were used as cooling off zones. In the cities, trees lined the streets, but the new urban world of the 60's was a commercial and financial world with high rise buildings, sealed central air systems and no fresh air.

The workers and the bosses were moving to the suburbs. The auto industry in Detroit had finally been able to make the drive home more pleasant with the development of the automobile air conditioner. Little by little, particularly in the hot, humid areas of the East and Midwest, the car with its windows rolled up on a summer day was the sign of a person with money (and comfort,) and everyone wanted to portray that image.

At the same time, the appliance manufacturers were marketing the window-mounted air conditioner. Naturally, these became necessary because after working in an air-conditioned office and driving home in the air-conditioned car, one wanted the same comfort at home. Now the new conversation revolved around the BTU rating of the window unit. The higher the BTU the more powerful the cooling capacity.

But, in the blink of an eye a new product made its debut on the market. This new product would satisfy the needs of the hot, humid world of the Midwest, the South as well as the folks in the Northeast. This wonder product was the Central Air Conditioner. Now the home was on the same level as the office. No more ugly window unit(s) marring the House Beautiful exterior. Central Air was a requirement of the rising middle class.

By the end of the 60's, the modern homeowner had central heating AND central air conditioning. The homeowner also had two automobiles with heating and air conditioning, getting an average 12-14 miles per gallon of fuel. On an average day, no one in the United States was outdoors except to walk to the car, which was now occupying a room of its own called an *attached garage.*

Of course, there was outdoor exposure from the car to the office or factory. The wife still had to face fresh, clean outdoor air from the parking lot at the supermarket, the cleaners, the drugstore and so on, in order to do the necessary shopping and errand running. Even the kids were getting less fresh air, namely because of television which pretty well assured their after school activity to be indoors.

In short, we were now living in enclosed environments with the occasional exceptions of attending a baseball game, a picnic, going to the swimming pool, taking in a drive-in movie, an autumn football game, or some other outdoor function preferably attended in the spring or fall. Indeed vacations, though still outdoor oriented for many, were for the most, another indoor activity, except when waiting in line for the next ride at Disneyland or Six Flags.

Despite the withdrawal into the cocoon of the modern home, the cheap cost of power had not forced the contractors to completely seal homes up and therefore, most of our homes still "breathed." This was about to change.

In the process of this change, people across America would find themselves exposed to an entire new set of problems. Particularly when it came to all of the materials used in the construction of their homes. Now, with the modern methods of construction, the uses of synthetics for nearly everything from floor to ceiling, and the furnishings in-between, it's no wonder that problems would begin to arise.

In 1973, OPEC decided it should be getting more money for its oil. The major Arab oil producers, along with the Shah of Iran, decided they wanted to be wealthier. The squeeze began and soon oil prices rose to impressive heights (remember odd-even day gas lines?) Not only did oil prices rise; supplies were reduced particularly to the United States. After the scramble to deal with gasoline prices and supplies, it became clear that the price of electricity would also rise. The same with heating oil, although heating oil remains in use around the country, albeit with much more efficiency than the systems of the 1950's and 1960's.

The winter of 1973 came and with it a horrifying sense of what it was going to cost to heat a home to a cozy temperature. This time the topic of conversation was the thermostat setting at home and in the office. Soon every office displayed a clear acrylic box locked over the thermostat and we all learned about the method of layered clothing when dressing. Conversations were soon returned to "R" factors and double paned windows gave way to triple paned windows.

The mixture of seeking comfort for 30 years (from the 50's through the 80's), building homes and offices for comfort, creating appliances for comfort, all this was going down the tube. The new focus was to be Energy Efficient.

Somewhere under the state of Louisiana, the government began storing a huge stockpile of crude oil to support the establishment of purported *energy independence*. Not only was the United States going to be Energy Independent, every appliance was to have increased energy efficiency thereby conserving much more energy.

Stoves, ovens, refrigerators, hot water heaters, washers, dryers, central heat and air conditioners were all emblazoned with yellow tags or stickers informing us what it would cost to operate any of these appliances and how energy efficient they are.

Had there actually been a true breakthrough in achieving greater efficiency? A careful comparison disproves that marketing ploy. What had been achieved was the use of yellow tags and stickers plastered on expensive appliances. Along with promotion of energy efficiency came the nearly evangelistic cry for Energy Conservation. Across the country there arose a new brand of advocates, decrying the very use of any energy whatsoever! The oil crisis merely served as a lubricant for this group of people to make their attacks on coal and nuclear power sources believable, at the same time and in the same breath.

This new Return to Nature mentality resulted in the meteoric sales of wood-burning stoves. Across the country little metal chimneys popped up through roofs. It looked like a 'Lil Abner comic depiction of Appalachian places like "Skunk Hollow." The only thing missing was the outhouse. Considering the air pollution inside this Back to Nature environment, the outhouse would have at least afforded the residents some moments of fresh air.

As a result, many wood burning stoves, with their cute little chimneys were not being installed safely or correctly, the movement of wood burning stoves was slowed somewhat because homes were burning in a conflagration of fire and/or releasing dangerous toxic fumes into the atmosphere. It wasn't long before we came to realize that entire areas were being blanketed with thick smoke. This brought back memories of the soft coal furnaces and their yellow pall of smoke.

Local Air Quality agencies tried to clamp down. However, exclusions were allowed, IF the wood stove was the sole source of heat. Regrettably, many citizens lied and received exemptions.

Ten years after the 1973 Oil Crisis, homes in the United States were being built and sold as Energy Efficient. Local ordinances were changed to force this new and supposedly correct way to create a dwelling. Homes being remodeled were caught in these new regulations as well. The new regulations cost thousands of extra dollars. Many people simply could not afford to make improvements due to the added expense.

Homebuilders made it sound as if the new codes would result in higher prices, although builders did little or nothing to fight these so-called Energy Conservation measures. Why? Actually these new codes saved/made them money. They charged more under the pretext that the new codes were costly to carry out.

The new codes set up ratios between square footage of living space and window area. This reduced the number of windows and/or the size of windows to be installed. Now came the Thermopane type window, or if you wanted to pay more, there was the triple pane window. The air spaces were not called "dead air spaces" anymore. They were filled with Argon or some other exotic gas.

Many windows did not open, again reducing the costs. The new insulation standard, not quite as onerous as touted, *but* for added cost you could upgrade the "R factor." Sealing the house with Tyvek or any similar synthetic wrapper, as well as caulking around windows, doors and every hole in the drywall, such as electric receptacles, outlets and switches, as well as holes through which pipes enter the house, made the new homes even less able to "breathe." We were now creating virtually airtight dwellings. Our homes could no longer "breathe."

To reduce the effects of accumulated moisture, which is the culprit in creating mildew, molds, bacteria, viruses and a myriad of other unhealthy effects of this air-tightness, the addition of Air Venting Fans was the supposed solution. On the wall, there appeared small contraptions looking like that joke of a fan that has graced bathroom ceilings since modern builders decided *no one needed a window in the bathroom!* For decades that window made bathrooms a tolerable habitat. The window, which is so necessary for fresh air, had been replaced with the exhaust fan. Often the noisy exhaust fan is absolutely useless in purging the odors and moisture associated with this room.

While on the subject of the bathroom, a bigger farce is that the exhaust fans do not normally exhaust to the outside. Nearly all exhaust into the attic or overhead spaces in a home.

These little air venting fans (look closely at one sometime) were now gracing the walls and attempted to remove foul, moist air from the now sealed living spaces. Did they work? Come on, folks. Think about it. The house is built airtight. The heating and cooling units, depending on the weather, do not have to do anything other than keep recirculating foul, humid air of your interior air space at the temperature you have selected. If air tightness is the result of this effort, then how is a little vent fan actually going to achieve the desired effect?

If it is going to work, then it has to have one hole, or a series of holes having access to new air, equal to the capacity of the exhaust fan. Then new air can flow in to purge the old air from the living areas.

The question really boils down to how fast you want this change of air to occur, and at what point. It depends on the power of the fan and of course, you still have to have an inlet of new air from the outside.

The typical living room of say, 25 feet x 35 feet with 8-foot ceilings has a volume of 7000 cubic feet (which is considered the norm). If you want new air to replace the old stale air every hour, then a vent fan is required to freely exhaust 116 cubic feet per minute. The key word here is *freely*, meaning there is an inflow of new air from some source, be it a vent or a window opened enough to equal the capacity of the exhaust fan(s).

Some folks have spent money installing heat exchangers. These units remove the old air and, as they exhaust it, the heat from the old air is transferred to the incoming fresh air. The same process occurs with outgoing cool air transferring the coolness to the incoming warm air. These units are not cheap. Apparently, they have arguable economic efficiency.

A question that has piqued curiosity throughout the evolution of comfort in the home, and the attempt to make homes supposedly more energy efficient, is why have homes gotten so much larger? Doesn't the very term, *energy efficient* bring to mind something that would contribute to the conservation of energy? Building Energy Efficient was supposed to reduce the homeowner's cost. However, in reality, it has only made the providers of energy wealthier.

In the 60's, a 2200 square foot home was considered to be quite luxurious. In the 70's, 2500 to 2700 square feet was typical of the upscale house. Now, even retired people buy very upscale homes of 4000 square feet. Their offspring, who can afford a home, seem to think nothing of 4000 to 5000 square feet or more as a moderately upscale dwelling.

Reason and logic dictate that despite oil crisis alleged conservation efforts and so-called improvements in efficiency in the building of homes, nothing has been really saved. However, on the contrary, home prices have increased as well as the size of homes. The cost to achieve comfort in these airtight domiciles has increased likewise.

Something far more serious has occurred in the process of creating these airtight, efficient, energy conserving, devourers of cash. In our technological genius, we have created living spaces, which can more aptly be called *killing spaces*. The children growing up in these airtight, energy efficient homes are paying a horrendous price with respect to their health and well-being. In many instances, so are their parents.

The preceding pages are offered as a brief sketch of today's many commonplace elements, which whether we like it or not, have become an

9-OCON

everyday component of our living spaces. Whether that living space is located in an apartment, a cooperative, a condo, townhouse, suburban home, a country estate or a vacation hideaway. They are all similar in the materials, appliances, and so-called energy conservation efforts.

CHAPTER 2

THE CHEMICALLY TOXIC HOME

Let's return to the dwellings we live in so we can learn the hazards they hold for our family's health and ourselves. The structures we erect to use as dwelling spaces all really commence at the government agencies that issue the permits to build. With money in hand and the plans for the proposed dwelling space, one goes before these government minions to literally ask permission to begin. It is at this point, when modern dwellings and those being refurbished begin to be made unhealthy.

It is here that the window space to floor space ratios are assured. The minimums are the goal. From ventilation to potential energy consumption, all are forced to illogical minimums.

Naturally, any attempt to deviate from their codebooks is nearly catastrophic. To seek alternatives or develop common sense compromises (which might yield a healthier home) is absolutely tantamount to committing treason. This situation is the result of politicians, who generally

9-OCON

have no experience or knowledge of construction, yet pass laws that the building permit people are stuck with enforcing. We can't blame them.

EXCAVATION: This is the first act that institutes the process of opening the Pandora's box of bacteria, viruses, microbes and other germs that inhabit the soil. To say nothing of the many other toxic chemicals and God only knows what, that lie beneath the soil.

Nearly any house will require some level of excavation, depending upon the terrain and climatic conditions. The type of foundation used makes a big difference. If you are putting a home on a slab, this can usually require the least amount of earth movement, but it can also create bigger problems. Homes with a crawl space and raised foundation usually require more earth movement. Of course, the homes built on a basement space or daylight basement require the largest amount of earth movement. In the process of each of these excavations, serious problems are created which can affect your health and the health of your family, now and in the future.

THE SLAB: This is simply a reinforced concrete slab poured on a prepared base of crushed rock or sand. Footings are part of the slab. This is known as a MONOLITH type slab, used in the mildest and drier climates. Another type is the floating slab. This is used where soils are not stable, or where moisture or frost levels are a factor. It is composed of formed footings. Concrete is poured between the footings once they have set.

How could these slabs be a future health problem? The answer is fairly uncomplicated. Despite reinforcing concrete slabs crack. They may be hairline cracks or fairly noticeable cracks. Even with visqueen vapor barriers put down between the prepared bed and the slab, these cracks will allow moisture to migrate through them. Plus, for some reason, concrete just loves to act as a wick drawing moisture up through the concrete cracks causing untold problems such as deadly molds, mildew and fungus. Therefore, most have their usefulness compromised when the concrete is poured and the sharp edges of rock and other materials cause punctures in the plastic vapor barrier.

However, moisture is not the only invader. With the passage of time ants and termites can work their way into these cracks and eventually into the home. If cracks and moisture provide critters as big an ant access, the question is what can enter that you can't see? Did anyone see what was in the topsoil and below the soil's surface? Microbes from some long forgotten dump or chemicals from decades ago? Environmental concerns are a relatively new thinking process. In the years past, it was not unusual for folks to dump any number of toxic wastes on the ground. This remains a common practice today with perhaps the exception that now it is hidden when it is covered with soil. It is this stuff that can also enter your home through those insignificant cracks in a slab foundation.

THE REGULAR FOOTING FOUNDATION: This is the most common foundation found throughout the country. It has been around awhile, so older homes and new construction sit atop this foundation.

If you were of a mind to design a really dark, damp habitat for every kind of spore, microbe and any other visible and invisible source of potential health hazards, this is it. This incubator of an unhealthy stew is popularly known as a *crawl space*. One enters this space by doing several body-beating gyrations. This gives you the opportunity to practice being in the army infantry or a circus acrobat! Trying to crawl is sometimes possible, but usually you are on your back or your stomach. If your home is insulated, you get to enjoy dust and fiberglass on your face, in your eyes, and anywhere your clothing and your skin come into contact. Also worth mentioning are the spiders and other mini creatures residing here, both seen and unseen. Many of these crawl spaces will have a layer of plastic on the surface. Quite possibly an attempt was made to tack another plastic vapor barrier underneath the floor which forces the toxic gases upward into your living space. Nonetheless, the moisture is all around and more than likely will also find its way up into your home.

It's really too bad builders and buyers won't spend a few hundred dollars more to concrete these crawl space floors and put a drain at a low point. This would do a great deal to make the space more accessible.

THE BASEMENT OR DAYLIGHT BASEMENT: In many areas of the country the basement is a part of life. Before refrigeration they were known as cellars and served as a cool storage area. In hot or cold weather they served as a place to play, do the laundry and for storage. One thing they all had in common was a lot of dampness. This dampness obviously influences the growth of toxic molds and fungus. Today even with better materials to seal out moisture, basements are damp and without lighting, they are dark. Many are dug deep enough to require a sump pump to keep them from becoming under-house pools. For violent weather such as tornadoes or hurricanes they are extremely useful, but otherwise most basements serve as a damp, dark incubator for all sorts of dangerous life forms.

The daylight basement is only slightly different in design. Usually one of its sides is at ground level but the other three walls and the floor still afford moisture an opportunity to introduce itself into the living spaces to produce the life threatening toxic molds and fungus.

So, whether your home is atop a slab, a footing with a crawl space or some form of basement, the potential for future unhealthy conditions are a reality and eventually can invade the living space.

THE WALLS, ROOF AND SUB-FLOORS: The slab foundation is ready for walls, roof trusses and sheathing. We'll return to the sheathing later. Those homes built on footings or basements use floor joists and a sub-floor. In the past, floor joists were 2 x 10's or 12's on 12-inch centers. Today we use the glue and wood chips pressed into a sheet, and glue (2) 2"x2"s, one on each side, and call it an engineered floor joist. Once upon a long time ago, the sub-floors were 7/8-inch tongue-in-groove natural woods. Again, glued and smashed wood chip sheets are used as sub-floors. These engineered sub-floors are giving off degassing vapors for months or years. In addition, the numerous glues and adhesives used in the construction may take years to degas.

This same glue and wood chip sheathing is what covers your outside walls and roof. To assure your home is airtight, and to keep the sheathing dry, the outside walls are covered with yet another petroleum based product, tarpaper or Tyvek. Therefore, the glue in the sheathing can only degas to the interior through and around the soon to be installed fiberglass insulation and drywall.

Once the roofing materials are in place and the windows set, the house is *"weathered in,"* meaning the interior of the house is able to remain dry if it rains. The house, despite the tarpaper or the Tyvek wrapping, is still a fairly benign place. But, that will change soon enough.

Once the plumber and electrician have finished their *"rough in"* piping and wiring, along come the heating and air-conditioning team installing the ducts and vents to keep you comfortable, or so they believe. When this is completed, the insulation arrives. The installers proceed to roll, stuff and cram itchy fiberglass insulation into every nook and cranny. The drywall hangers finish this sealing process. Essentially, your home has now become a cocoon, or a tomb, depending upon how you view sealed spaces.

From this point forward, we commence mixing the chemical soup that will affect you and your family the most in the beginning. As the house slowly becomes colonized by other interesting and potentially malign life-forms and their waste products, as well as your own, plus the introductions you and your family bring in from other places, our toxic soup is now a hodge-podge.

First, the walls are coated with a primer, then paint. Of course, many will opt for some texture on the walls and ceiling. By and large, the *"cottage cheese"* is a thing of the past. It was an overhead jungle of dust, mites and spores of every kind.

It is the wall textures, which still offer literally millions of great footholds for all sorts of life forms, dust and pollens. Until you repaint, those walls are the safest places for anything to attach itself or be attached. If wallpaper is used as a wall covering, you now have moisture absorbing material that not only serves to enhance mold and spore production, but also creates a space between the wallpaper and the drywall and, to top it off, the paste used to attach the wall paper is often wheat based which helps in the nutrition of these living organisms as well as growing its own variety of fungi.

FORMALDEHYDE: Formaldehyde is an important chemical used widely by industry to manufacture building materials and numerous household products. It is also a by-product of combustion and certain other natural processes. Thus, it may be present in substantial concentrations both indoors and outdoors.

Sources of formaldehyde in the home include building materials, smoking, household products, and the use of unvented, fuel-burning appliances, like gas stoves or kerosene space heaters. Formaldehyde, by itself or in combination with other chemicals, serves a number of purposes in manufactured products. For example, it is used to add permanent-press qualities to clothing and draperies, as a component of glues and adhesives, and as a preservative in some paints and coating products.

In homes, the most significant sources of formaldehyde are likely to be pressed wood products made using adhesives that contain urea-formaldehyde (UF) resins. Pressed wood products made for indoor use include: particleboard (used as subflooring and shelving and in cabinetry and furniture); hardwood plywood paneling (used for decorative wall covering and used in cabinets and furniture); and medium density fiberboard (used for drawer fronts, cabinets, and furniture tops.) Medium density fiberboard contains a higher resin-to-wood ratio than any other UF pressed wood product and is generally recognized as being the highest formaldehyde-emitting pressed wood product.

Other pressed wood products, such as softwood and flake or oriented strand board, are produced for exterior construction use and contain the dark, or red/black-colored phenol-formaldehyde (PF) resin. Although formaldehyde is present in both types of resins, pressed woods that contain PF resins generally emit formaldehyde at considerably lower rates than those containing UF resin.

Since 1985, The Department of Housing and Urban Development (HUD) has permitted only the use of plywood and particleboard that conform to specified formaldehyde emission limits in the construction of prefabricated and mobile homes. In the past, some of these homes had elevated levels of formaldehyde because of the large amount of high-emitting pressed wood products used in their construction and because of their relatively small interior space.

The rate at which products like pressed wood or textiles release formaldehyde can change. Formaldehyde emissions will generally decrease as products age. When the products are new, high indoor temperatures or humidity can cause increased release of formaldehyde from these products.

During the 1970's, many homeowners had urea-formaldehyde foam insulation (UFFI) installed in the wall cavities of their homes as an energy conservation measure. However, many of these homes were found to have relatively high indoor concentrations of formaldehyde soon after the UFFI installation. Few homes are now being insulated with this product. Studies show that formaldehyde emissions from UFFI decline with time; therefore, homes in which UFFI was installed many years ago may not have high levels of formaldehyde now.

HEALTH EFFECTS OF FORMALDEHYDE—Formaldehyde, a colorless, pungent-smelling gas, can cause watery eyes, burning sensations in the eyes and throat, nausea, and difficulty in breathing in some humans exposed at elevated levels (above 0.1 parts per million.) High concentrations may trigger attacks in people with asthma. There is evidence that some people can develop sensitivity to formaldehyde. It has also been shown to cause cancer in animals and may cause cancer in humans.

MAINTAIN MODERATE TEMPERATURE AND HUMIDITY LEVELS AND PROVIDE ADEQUATE VENTILATION.

The rate at which formaldehyde is released is accelerated by heat and may also depend somewhat on the humidity level. Therefore, the use of dehumidifiers and air conditioning to control humidity and to maintain a moderate temperature can help reduce formaldehyde emissions. (Drain and clean humidifier collection trays frequently so that they do not become a breeding ground for microorganisms.) Increasing the rate of ventilation in your home will also help in reducing formaldehyde levels.

SOURCES: Pressed wood products (hardwood plywood wall paneling, particleboard, fiberboard) and furniture made with these pressed wood products. Urea-formaldehyde foam insulation (UFFI.) Combustion sources and environmental tobacco smoke. Durable press drapes, other textiles, and glues.

HEALTH EFFECTS: Eye, nose, and throat irritation; wheezing and coughing; fatigue; skin rash; severe allergic reactions. May cause cancer. May also cause other effects listed under "organic gasses."

LEVELS IN HOME: Average concentrations in older homes without UFFI are generally well below 0.1 (ppm.) In homes with significant amounts of new pressed wood products, levels can be greater than 0.3 ppm.

STEPS TO REDUCE EXPOSURE:

- Use "exterior-grade" pressed wood products (lower-emitting because they contain phenol resins, not urea resins.)
- Use air conditioning and dehumidifiers to maintain moderate temperature and reduce humidity levels.

- Increase ventilation, particularly after bringing new sources of formaldehyde into the home.

To a certain degree, the acrylic and latex paints currently used are still toxic. They all use silica as filler. So, if one needs to sand it, it will introduce silica into the living space where it will remain as a lung irritant. We should not forget that many of these coatings contain ethylene glycol, or *antifreeze*.

In most instances, the sub-floor is formulated from sawdust and formaldehyde, and glues. The same potentially toxic glues are used for the wall and roof sheathing. Since the house has been wrapped for air tightness, these glues will continue to degas long after they are cured. This process of degassing may take months or years. The degassing process can actually increase if moisture levels in the house are high. Moisture levels will be high because the house has been wrapped so airtight. The chemical mixtures used to make the sheathing and particleboard is formulated for interior use, but interiors are now experiencing much higher moisture levels.

With the installation of various interior cabinets we have another source of formaldehyde coatings and other glues combining to make the chemical soup even more toxic. Today, cabinets installed in kitchens, bathroom, and laundry rooms are generally prefabricated using particleboard and laminated with plastic. Every shelf and door is made with the material. In the bathrooms, sinks, tubs, showers and their surrounds are manufactured using "cultured stone" which are combinations of polyester resins, limestone and other ground stone powders simulating marble, granite or rock. Corian and other similar cabinet tops and work surfaces are made from these resins. Although these materials take hours to cure, the gases resulting from the catalytic actions will continue to be released for months, or years.

Closet doors throughout the house may be formed of Masonite, a chemical mix of chemicals like formaldehyde, glues and paper or wood mix.

Many are now made of formed styrene plastic, which will continue to degas for years and if exposed to sunlight, will eventually decompose. Trim molding, etc. are too often urethane foam with a plastic coating. Paneling will be composed of highly toxic toluene and methyl ethyl ketone based contact cements.

The last of the ingredients going into our chemical soup are the floor coverings. The no-wax designer vinyl floor covering used in kitchens and bathrooms are composed of materials that can cause allergic reactions. However, the real villain in the floor-covering category is the carpet along with the pad underneath. These two materials degas a chemical soup that includes formaldehyde and numerous other petroleum based chemical colorants and synthetics used to create the fiber, as well as the backing and glues. Degassing can include formaldehyde, toluene (which is known to cause birth defects and reproductive harm) and xylene (which may affect the brain and nervous system causing dizziness, headache or nausea). Other chemicals may include methyl methacylate, ethyl benzine, methylene and naphthalene. The least offensive of any carpet is synthetic untreated nylon on jute backing, or cotton or wool if using natural fibers.

The following is a list of the most common chemical vapor sources in remodeled and new home construction. Although this is just a short list of noxious, toxic and hazardous materials that are taken for granted by us all, nonetheless, they are just as perilous as pointing a loaded gun at your head.

METHYL ETHYL KETONE (M.E.K.)
Contains Petroleum Distillate. Flammable. *KEEP OUT OF REACH OF CHILDREN.*
Used for thinning, cleaning fiberglass resins epoxies vinyl, lacquers and adhesives.

LOCTITE
Stick 'n Seal adhesive: Contains toluene and hexane. Avoid breathing vapors.

HOWARD PRODUCTS WOOD STAIN:
Contains Toluene and xylene. Petroleum distillates. May be fatal if swallowed or inhaled. A little goes a long way.

LACQUER THINNER;
Contains petroleum distillate. Methanol, toluene, acetone, methyl ethyl ketone, propylene glycol, monomethyl ether acetate, ethyl acetate and rylene. Vapor harmful. Extremely flammable
SPECIAL WARNING: Exposure to toluene is known to cause birth defects or reproductive harm. Talk about a cocktail!

NYBCO SPRAY PAINT:
SPECIAL WARNING: Contains toluene, acetone and petroleum distillates. Vapor harmful. May affect the brain or nervous system causing dizziness, headache or nausea. Causes eye, nose, throat and skin irritation.

RAMUC PAINT (Butyl alcohol):
Contains xylene, methyl isobutyl, and ketone. Vapor harmful. May affect the brain or nervous system causing dizziness, headache or nausea. Causes eye, nose, throat and skin irritation. May be harmful when absorbed through the skin.

RAINBUSTER 345 CONTRACTOR GRADE: 23 tubes (30 fl. oz. each) 2400 sq. ft. home. This product is used in new home construction subfloors to prevent squeaky floors.

Contains calcium carbonate 1317-65-3, Ethyl Benzene 100-41-4, Methylene Bisphenyl Isocyanate 101-68-8, Titanium Dioxide 13463-67-7, Xylene 1330-20-7.

This product contains the following listed chemicals known to the state of California to cause cancer, birth defects or other reproductive harm: Di

(2 Ethylhexyl) Phithalate, Nickel, and vinyl chloride. Volatile Organic Compounds, which may cause allergic skin and eye, burns.

CLEAR SILICONE

(Caulk) Releases Acetic acid.

GEOCEL (2000) CONSTRUCTION CAULKING SEALANT:

CAUTION: Contains PMacetate CAS# 108-85-6 and "aromatic" hydro-carbons CA5 64742-85-6. Harmful or fatal if swallowed. Harmful if inhaled within a closed area. Avoid skin contact.

QUAD ADVANCED FORMULA SEALANT:

Contains mineral spirits and Xylene. Exposure to vapors may cause respiratory tract problems, headaches and dizziness and is anesthetic.

OATEY PLASTIC PIPE GLUE:

DANGER vapors harmful. May be absorbed through skin. Acetone-Methyl Ethyl Ketone. Cycloheranone 108-94-1 and tetrahydrofuron 109-99-9.

ATCO AMERICAN TAR COMPANY (RAIN SEAL) 1821:

WARNING: Contains petroleum distillates. Harmful or fatal if swallowed. Clean tools with paint thinner. (i.e. see Lacquer thinner)

PPG EPOXY PRIMER CATALYST:

Contains amine, alcohols, glycol ethers, ketones, xylene, toluene, esters, resins #. Photochemically reactive.

ANTIBACTERIAL KITCHEN CLEANERS: Keep out of Reach of Children.

Contains dimethyl benzyl ammonium chlorides. Precautionary Statements: Hazards to human and domestic animals. CAUTION: May cause eye irritation.

3M SUPER 77 SPRAY ADHESIVE AEROSOL ADHESIVE (used in drywall taping process)

Contains cyclohexane 110-82-7, methylpentane 107-83-5, demethylether 11-10-6, isobutane 75-28-5, propane 74-98-6, 3 methylpentane 96-14-0, 2,3 dimethylbutane 7-229-8, 2 dimethylbutane 75-83-2 and N-hexane 110-54-3.

KRYLON, MYBCO & RUST/OLIUM SPRAY PAINTS
Contain acetone, toluene, xylene and ketones

GOLDEN SPIKE SUB FLOOR ADHESIVE
Contains petroleum distillates, toluene and ethyl alcohol. Vapors are irritating to eyes and respiratory tract and cause headaches, dizziness and is anesthetic.

M-D SUB FLOOR ADHESIVE
Calcium carbonate, clay, synthetic rubber, toluene and VOC374GL.
WARNING: this product contains a chemical known to the State of California to cause cancer, birth defects or other reproductive harm.

PARKER WALL KOLOR Interior wall paint, thick & creamy

INGREDIENTS
Water	7732-18-5
Ethylene Glycol	- 107-21-1
Titanium Dioxide slurry	13463-67-7
Polyvinyl Acetate polymer	108-05-5
Hydrous Aluminate Silicate	1332-58-7
Calcium Carbonate	471-34-1

CAUTION: Avoid prolonged breathing of vapors and prolonged contact with skin.

THE ABOVE ARE BUT A FEW OF THE MATERIALS USED IN NEW CONSTRUCTION. THEY MAY ALSO BE USED IN REMODELING AN OLDER HOME.

Generally, most people take the warnings lightly or as empty statements because they do not recognize the chemical ingredients listed. However, if you are pregnant or planning a family, take heed. Read and understand the warnings listed.

The EPA has identified at least 3,000 indoor pollutants, a seemingly long list of potential dangers to you and your family. The question is; what can you do about the problem? It is not feasible to take the house apart and remove the guilty products. However, it is possible to alleviate the dangers of these vapors and, in the process, shorten the length of time during which they pose the greatest hazards.

As these products cure and age the emissions of vapors should slowly decrease. It is in the early application stages and the curing process when degassing, toxic vapor emissions are the highest. Depending on the product or material, this early, most active vapor emission period can vary from weeks to months and sometimes even years. The sooner you can counteract this early and highest emission toxic output, the better.

The simplest and most effective way to achieve this result is to know how to deal with the chemicals. If the chemicals degassing are exposed to controlled amounts of *super-charged oxygen*, (a definition given ozone by the Grolier Book of Popular Science as early as 1963), (O_3)/Ozone, the dangerous toxic gasses will be destroyed. The source of the ozone is the critical factor. Here one wants to rely only on pure ozone created with very specific ultraviolet light. For a new or remodeled home, a treatment once every 3 to 4 months will rapidly reduce the danger of emissions in the home and consequently, the net amount of toxic vapors in the air. After 3 or 4 treatments the problems associated with harmful vapor emissions will drop dramatically in most circumstances.

The most exciting and satisfying outcome using the super-charged oxygen method is the wonderful sense of well being which you will experience, knowing your family has a healthy and healthful environment in which to enjoy the efforts of your labor, love and concern. Don't ever overlook the simple fact that your efforts today will be remembered when your children are making the same wise decision for their families, your grandchildren.

We have a lot more to cover in this book. Before we move on, I would like to make an observation. Since you are still reading this book, I have to believe you are interested in the problems of the *sick home syndrome*. Quite possibly you have read newspaper or magazine articles regarding this problem and realize this is a factual and growing menace to everyone's health and well-being. Obviously, you are interested in defending your home and family against this threat. It is a person like yourself, one who has a sincere commitment to his family, their health and future, and who may realize that not only is there a huge number of families with similar concerns but who also need to have their future and health protected.

You may be someone who would enjoy a challenging and certainly meaningful new career, or to enhance an existing profession or business. If any of this has struck a cord or stimulated some interest, please call 425-672-4808.

9-OCON

CHAPTER 3

BIOLOGICAL WARFARE IN THE HOME

50% of homes contain problem molds
A new study attributes nearly 100% of chronic sinus infections to mold
A 300% increase in the asthma rate over the past 20 years has been
linked to mold

THE REAL CULPRIT

Considering all the chemicals used in the construction and completion
of a home, there remains a very undeniable problem and that is the bacteria, viruses, spores, molds, fungi and pollens that begin inhabiting a
home as it is under construction and continue to propagate. We make the
environment and existence of these potential toxic enemies easier by
reducing fresh air ventilation. This reduction increases the humidity con-
tent. Not only do we provide the perfect state of damp air environment,
but with dirty filters in vent systems and dirty air ducts, we actually grow
our own hybrids and mutants. We mix and stir this cellular soup with

wonderful biological blenders such as vacuum cleaners, fans, central heating and air conditioning. We also provide great gardens for the hatching, germinating, reproduction and overall success of every kind of microbe, germ, virus, bacteria, spore, mite, fungus and so on, with wall-to-wall carpet. That wall-to-wall carpet can hold up to 10,000,000 organisms in a square foot alone!

DUST MITES AND THEIR FECES

If you are creating ideal conditions for the many life forms that will get to be your closest companions, then you really ought to get to know them. Nothing worse than throwing a party and the guests are strangers. Who are the unwanted guests? What attracts them? What makes them stay and how do you get rid of them?

Many people are aware of the little critter called a dust mite. These are microscopic insects that live in dust. They particularly like fabric, carpets, pillows, upholstered furniture and stuffed animals. They thrive in this cozy warmth and humidity thus enhancing their reproduction. The highest concentrations of these mites are now found in so-called "energy efficient" homes. Of the 35 million Americans suffering from allergies, the majority suffer from dust mites in their own home, along with other home allergens rather than the typical summer hay fever and pollen sources that are no less miserable to endure.

The dust mite is not itself the culprit. The mite feeds on shed human skin scales. We all produce skin scales as our outer, or epidermal, skin layer sloughs off and is replenished by living layers beneath. The outer epidermal layer, or stratum corneum, is formed from several layers of flattened cells that become horny, have lost their nuclei and contain keratin. Everyday this outer layer falls off or is shed. The mites eat this dead skin. However, the allergic reaction comes from the *feces* of the dust mite that cause the problems.

Dust mites are a fact of life. However, there are some remedies that can be utilized to eliminate dust mites and will go a long way in reducing their numbers and their output of the allergy causing feces they produce.

FUNGUS

Molds, mildews, yeasts and mushrooms are all fungi, which must feed off other organic material, particularly decaying matter. But for this decaying matter to be consumed by fungi there has to be some moisture. In short, fungi love homes with excess humidity. They flourish in the modern "energy efficient" home as well as older homes with moisture in all the wrong places. The real threat from fungi is the millions of spores released into the air, their means of reproduction and survival.

There are thousands of forms of fungi. However, in the home there are usually only a few dozen. The majorities are molds and mildews. Mold is usually identified as a downy or furry growth. Mildew is usually seen as a thin, furry coating, often whitish in color.

It is those little spores coming from these organisms that wreak the real havoc. They are, on average, about one micron in size (1 micron = .000039 inch). That's very small. So small, in fact, that it takes 25,000 all in a row to equal 1 inch. These spores cause everything from itchy eyes, to fatigue, bronchitis, allergic rhinitis, as well as asthma.

Fungus living in the house finds a large selection of material from which to feed. Fungi will feed off petroleum products found in paints, wall paper, gases in the air, kitchen residue, laundry hampers, damp shoes, carpeting, carpet padding, wicker furniture. Wicker baskets are also great feeding grounds. Old books, magazines, and some types of caulking used around bathtubs and showers can be home to many different fungi.

With these varied food sources, the other necessary ingredient is moisture. Make sure the laundry dryer vents are clean and that the dryer properly vents to the outside. The moisture added by cooking, bathing, and dishwashing all act to stimulate fungus growth, which in turn causes more spore production, thus creating a productive, toxic garden. In addition, each family member adds several gallons of water per person, per day as a result of respiration and perspiration. Another very excellent source of nourishment for fungi and mold spores are humidifiers. Allowing standing water in these units for any period of time is a source for fungi and mold growth.

HUMIDITY IN THE HOME

A certain amount of humidity in the home is desirable for health and comfort. But too much moisture in the air increases the rate of incubation and mutations of fungi growth, encourages the production of toxic molds, smuts, mildew, yeasts, bacteria and viruses and also does the same for such things as dust mites. Ideally, a relative humidity level of 50% or less is the target zone for comfort. Higher levels result in creating excessive fungus contamination or dust mite production. To prevent microclimates in spaces such as closets, it is useful to use louvered closet doors and also to arrange furnishings to avoid dead air spaces.

Another excellent source of nourishment for fungi growth is the drip pan underneath a self-defrosting refrigerator and the water collection drip pan inside your air conditioner unit. Remember the Legionnaire's disease a few years back? The problem was finally isolated in the air conditioning system at the convention.

Another area of the home that contributes to fungi/mold spore production is the basement or crawl space. Both are excellent incubators for all the previously discussed nasty things simply because of the cooler, fluctuating temperatures that result in a higher relative humidity. Plus, both are often supplied with moisture from the ground or "rising damp" atmosphere. Even if the home has been *sealed* between the living area and these areas, the toxic spores produced will find their way inside.

Two other zones of the home have also become huge problem areas for fungi growth. These are the roof cavities and wall cavities. The use of insulation without considering moisture migration inside a house is beginning to prove a real health problem, and eventually a safety problem.

As moisture migrates through the wall and the insulation, it becomes cooler. As the moisture cools it begins to condense resulting in wet insulation and eventually, wet wood. The moisture causes the formaldehyde glues to deteriorate and degas. Many types of insulation, including foam, are composed of a formaldehyde type of ingredient. Additionally, the moisture begins to soak into the structural part of the house, and the process called "wood rot" begins. Of course, wood rot is again, a fungus, producing spores that along with mold and mildew growing in the insulation and on the backside of the drywall are all able to enter your home. The use of moisture barriers on the inside of the house, before drywall goes up, is supposed to stop this moisture migration. If anything, this barrier enhances the problem because, in some cases, it traps the moisture.

The moisture barrier concept has been part of the insulation theory for some time. Right behind this theory comes the "air barrier" theory, and it may actually be more important particularly with regard to the health of your family. The moisture barrier is susceptible to holes but can still function as a barrier. However, the "air tightness" theory requires 100% air tightness and causes a very real health threat.

Whatever the latest concept may be, in an effort to save a few dollars under the guise of energy costs, the bottom line is that homes have become nearly sealed tombs with barely enough fresh air to breath. Now fungi producing toxic molds and mildew can grow where they once never did, plus they are now combined with other numerous chemicals and residue gases your grandparents never heard of.

Never before has it been so crucial that a home be kept free of fungi and other living critters that actually do pose a health threat that in generations before were not a real threat. Fungi and dust mites are as old or older than we humans. They may serve a purpose, but, in today's sealed homes, they are a very serious threat.

As with dust mites, eradication of molds is the optimum solution. Destroying the source of fungi is the only way to stop spore, germ, parasite, bacteria and virus production. The optimum solution is to have the ability to kill the fungus once and for all so that they are unable to reproduce. We must be more vigilant. We are at war and at any time it is a question of to *whom* we are losing. In the August 30, 1999 article in the U.S. New & World Report magazine addressed *casualties in the germ war*. Quoting directly, "another resistant strain of common staph bacterium raised its ugly head. E Coli strains have mutated to the point that the medical community has warned all of us that they simply cannot stay ahead of this catastrophic threat."

What do you do? How do you stop this potential onslaught against your family and rid your home of toxic gasses, chemicals, and parasitic dust mites, along with dangerous molds, bacteria and viruses?

FROM SINUS INFECTIONS TO ASTHMA, NEW RESEARCH IDENTIFIED HOUSEHOLD MOLD AS THE CULPRIT (USA WEEKEND DEC. 3-5, 1999)

Stachybotrys atra (pronounced Stack-ee-BOT-RIS) is an especially lethal mold. It's part of a family of molds (others are *memnoniella and aspergillus versicolor*) that produce airborne toxins, called mycotoxins, that can cause serious breathing difficulties, memory and hearing loss, dizziness, flu like symptoms, and bleeding in the lungs. In 1996 and 1999 studies by Eckardt Johanning, M.C., of the Eastern New York Occupational and Environmental Health Center, people with prolonged exposure to mycotoxins from *stachybotrys* and other fungi experienced chronic fatigue, loss of balance, irritability, memory loss and difficulty speaking. "These were college graduates who had been functioning at a high level, and now they can't." Johanning says.

Fortunately, *stachybotrys* isn't found in homes as often as milder molds such as *cladosporium*, *pennicillium* and *alternaria*. Those are common, especially in damp states such as Texas, Louisiana, Florida and Oregon. Yet even they can cause health problems, including chronic sinus and respiratory infections and asthma. A 1999 Mayo Clinic study pegged nearly all the chronic sinus infections afflicting 37 million Americans to molds. Recent studies also have linked molds to the tripling of the asthma rate over the past 20 years.

How common are these molds? A 1994 Harvard University School of Public Health study of 10,000 homes in the United States and Canada found half had "conditions of water damage and mold associated with 50 to 100% increase in respiratory symptoms," says Harvard's Jack Spengler.

When molds grow, it's usually in damp places, behind walls and under floors, above ceiling tiles or behind shower walls—wherever there are wet cellulose materials they can feed on, such as wood, ceiling tiles, plasterboard, or accumulations of organic material inside air-conditioning and heating systems. Water is the key. Without it, molds can't get started, much less spread. But when water is left to sit for even 24 hours, common molds can take hold. If water continues to sit and areas become completely saturated, that's when a more lethal mold, such as *stachybotrys* can move in.

In Michigan, Wisconsin and Minnesota in the mid-1980, thousands of middle-income families fell ill when their homes developed mold problems. This year in New York City, 125 families at Henry Phipps Plaza South filed an $8 billion mold lawsuit against their landlord. And four years ago in Cleveland, *stachybotrys* growth from unrepaired storm damage was suspected of causing pulmonary hemorrhage in 14 children, killing two.

WHY NEW HOMES ARE MOLDIER

What's behind the sudden mold epidemic? Experts point to modern home design, including materials used, such as fake stucco (great mold food when wet); the way insulation can trap moisture behind walls; and the fact that today's homes, like office buildings, are more airtight, with air-conditioning and heating systems recirculating contaminated air. Families can go for months, even years, without knowing where their symptoms are coming from.

New houses are more prone to mold problems than older houses, but a bad leak in any house anywhere in the country can cause a mold problem if not properly taken care of. And what starts as a small mold problem can grow to consume a home.

Q: *What are some of the biological problems I should be concerned about?*

A: Molds, mildew, fungi, bacteria and dust mites are some of the main biological pollutants inside the house. Some, such as pollen, are generated outside the home. Mold and mildew are generated in the home and release spores into the air. Mold, mildew, fungi and bacteria are often found in areas of the home that have high humidity levels, such as bathrooms, kitchens, laundry room or basements. Dust mites and animal dander are problematic when they become airborne during vacuuming, making beds or when textiles are disturbed.

Q: *What are some of the health effects?*

A: Allergic reactions are the most common health problems associated with biological pollutants. Symptoms often include watery eyes, runny nose and sneezing, nasal congestion, itching, coughing, wheezing and difficulty breathing, headache, dizziness and fatigue. Dust mites have been identified as the single most important trigger for asthma attacks.

Q: *How are biological contaminants transported through the house?*

A: Molds and dust mites thrive in areas of high humidity. Mold grows on organic materials such as paper, textiles, grease, dirt and soap scum. Mold spores float throughout the house, forming new colonies where they land. Dust mites thrive on dead human skin cells and in textiles such as bedding, carpeting and upholstery. When these textiles are disturbed during vacuuming, making beds or walking on carpet, the dust mite feces particles become airborne. Pollen, plant material that enters through windows or on pets, and animal dander also become airborne when disturbed. Infectious diseases caused by bacteria and viruses are generally passed from person to person through physical contact, but some circulate through indoor ventilation systems.

Concerned? I am. What can you do to prevent this biological warfare from debilitating you and your family? Once again we can turn to that too often overlooked but scientifically proven solution. It is time to go on the attack with supercharged oxygen, also known as ozone. The ozone we are talking about and using is the same naturally produced form of oxygen produced with ultraviolet light and not some potentially unnatural and/or potentially dangerous form of ozone.

We are using nature to fight this battle. All of the vile, health threatening biologicals, from dust mites and their feces to molds, mildew, viruses, fungi and bacteria are carbon based life forms, and as such they have a common enemy. That enemy is ozone.

When that unstable molecule of oxygen with 3 atoms of oxygen instead of 2, as found in the oxygen in the air, is released, it literally is on a search and destroy mission in order to shed that third atom of oxygen. Plus, as all things in Nature, it seeks to restore itself to balance, or to an oxygen molecule with 2 atoms.

As our 3-atom supercharged oxygen molecule finds any carbon-based combination, be it dust mites, feces, mold, mildew, fungi, viruses and other bacteria, it immediately releases that extra oxygen atom and the killing (oxidizing) process begins. That single oxygen atom attacks the organism's cells, literally blowing a hole in it and killing it. During a treatment millions of these attacks are occurring simultaneously throughout the zone treated. This is the solution. It is the most, if not only, means of winning this battle for you and your family's health, safety and well-being.

Once again, the reality of the threat is not imagined. It is very real. You and your friends, neighbors and your entire community is aware of the threat and dangers. You can solve the problem not only for your family but countless others. If such a challenge stimulates your mind, you might consider the potential of not only solving a very real and on-going problem, but also providing yourself with a rewarding and profitable career opportunity.

CHAPTER 4

CHEMICAL & BIOLOGICAL DANGERS AT THE DINNER TABLE

EATING RIGHT: THE NEWEST THREAT. . . . OR IS IT?

Though studying history has taken a back seat to computer literacy and video games, the truth of the matter is that history does repeat itself. When it comes to feeding yourself and your family the repetition of history is frighteningly uncanny.

Less than a century ago, investigative journalists began educating Americans on why their food was killing them. These journalists were called *muckrakers*. Although they investigated and exposed many levels of greed and corruption, it was their focus on the food industry that, for the next sixty or seventy years, allowed consumers to buy and eat food with confidence.

Prior to the turn-of-the-century, most Americans lived on farms or near enough to farm areas to be assured of fresh vegetables, meats, fruit and diary products. In the coastal areas, seafood was available, and the rivers provided fish. By the end of the First World War, the majority of Americans were living in the cities. The old farms were not so convenient. In stepped the food processors and purveyors. It was in this era that Borden, Swift, Kellogg, Post, Carnation, Heinz and others were born and thus began the modern food processing business.

The greed of these businessmen was very strong. It was not long before some very gutsy people, in the face of real harm and threats from these now revered names of the food business were able to get inside the slaughterhouses, the packinghouses, the mills and every level of the food processing business. What they found explained why people died, with great regularity, after consuming these various so-called processed food products. Some folks were sturdy enough to survive. Many others got very sick. Many of those who survived suffered for the rest of their lives.

After the exposure of the processing plants, the complete lack of sanitation, the mixing of everything from the floors and other contamination into the kettles, the U.S. government began to step in to inspect the processors and set basic guidelines and regulations for each phase of the processing of foods.

The stamp, *Inspected by USDA* actually came into being then. By the 40's, you could open soup cans and, not see the head or whole carcass of rats, mice, or insects. Catsup was made with real tomatoes, not pigments. The *free market* of the so-called entrepreneurs had been reined in and at least some control was being enforced. This will be necessary again in the near future, not only with our food supplies but every aspect of modern living that is now operated by the so-called "free market" better defined as the "greed market."

Federal and state inspectors patrolled food processors, took samples, enforced sanitary codes and fined or even shut down businesses that did not comply.

Throughout the 50's and into the late 70's, seldom did anyone worry about the quality of the food we were consuming. By the late 70's, we were controlling the use of certain pesticides. Research had forced many to be discarded as too toxic to the food chain. Higher costs made farms far more conscientious when it came to the use and application of pesticides.

Enter the 80's and now the repetition of history begins. With the rediscovery of the so-called "Market Economy" the security and quality of our food supplies began a long down hill slide. Federal inspections were reduced, as the government supposedly became more efficient and cost conscious. Many processors became responsible for self-regulation. Instead of *prevention*, the food processing business, along with the food service business, relied on a new method of assuring our safety. If we got sick or died, their insurance companies would handle the problem. Of course, major food contamination, especially if it causes major illness, still gets attention from the media, and then of course, we hear from our government (when it's too late) via a recall.

The final move that has virtually taken the subject of food safety controls back to the days of the muckrakers has been NAFTA (free trade) and with it, the internationalizing of the American food industry. These two factors have literally led to a situation that has begun to blow up in our faces.

A day does not pass where somewhere in the U.S. someone or many are stricken with some virulent biological. One day it's botulism, the next it's E. Coli or salmonella. The litany keeps growing. The excuses keep coming, but nobody has the courage to focus on the causes—the real causes. No one has had the courage to expose and communicate to the public the long-term effects of the produce coming into the grocery stores of America. Pesticides we have long outlawed here, but are still made by the same American companies and sold to American owned farm corporations in other countries, are applied by workers, harvested by them and their children and shipped to the U.S. for consumption by us all. The truth is that this is exactly what is happening every day. Any such whistle blowing about NAFTA and the whistle blower is no longer employed.

Whether it is grapes loaded with the residue of long since outlawed mercury based fungicides, strawberries with the same residue, or tomatoes harvested from fields with water coming from broken piping mixed with sewage, metallic and chemical runoff, we are at great risk.

Sounds like a description from the pages of the muckrakers. Well, it was exactly these conditions that prompted our food regulation laws. They were not perfect, but by and large they were effective most of the time. Not any more. Today, whether it is a trip to the market or grabbing a fast food special, you run far more risks than at anytime in the memorable past. You cannot even feel secure eating at an expensive restaurant. The most frightening scenario is the danger you face at home preparing what you believe to be a healthy meal, and the extra efforts you make to assure healthy snacks and liquid refreshments for your family. From a week-end lunch to an evening meal, today you run more risks of harming your family and friends than your great-grandparents faced on the farms of rural America before the advent of modern technical inventions such as hot running water and refrigeration.

Part of our inattention to these risks comes from the faith we still have, though without the same fervor, in the government's responsibility to protect our food supplies and us.

Over the past several years, the risks we face with something as basic as eating healthy food have reached serious levels. Whether your news comes from newspapers or the television, the mention of food related problems has increased and continues to do so with each and every passing day.

These reports are not just a few isolated incidents. On the contrary, many, if not most, of these are not reported. A good rule of thumb is that for every one you hear about there are thousands you do not. Even incidents in your own community are not all reported by local news media. Advertisers do not like to hear bad news about their products. The local Health Department may decide not to report such incidents for whatever reason. It seems as though the incident must involve serious or fatal consequences and/or the potential number of victims must be significant. These elements seem to be very influential for any state or federal notice.

But even with these factors affecting the true scope of the risks involved in the food supply system, something must be done and soon. Once again, the final responsibility for the health and safety of your family is yours.

THE NEW THREAT

Despite all of the talk over the past 20 years, the Environmental Protection Agency and Department of Agriculture have not hurt the farmers, or at least the few that are left. Nor have they intimidated the huge agribusiness companies that actually produce and supply the majority of the food in this country. The agri-business and the chemical companies are still using what they call *safe* and *acceptable* fungicides, miticides, insecticides, growth stimulators, growth retardants, insect sterilizers, hormones, weed controls and herbicides. All of which find their way into the food system. The EPA's biggest impact has been in the area of registering and labeling of this potentially toxic potpourri of modern chemistry. Whether labels are read and chemicals are properly applied is purely a guessing game. Even with bilingual labeling it is a question of one's ability in understanding the label.

We are talking about American produced food from the giant agri-business companies. Perhaps you are thinking that they must test for residues of these chemicals. Sure they do . . . at test sights run by either the government or the chemical companies with mixing and application done by, or strictly monitored by, trained scientists and similar personnel.

At the agri-business farm, the only concern is whether the amount used is within the budget allocated for that chemical. On the one hand, this sounds good (the old free market at work); the possibility of using too much chemical would be controlled by the cost. Not particularly true. If the crop is in trouble, extra expense to use more than the prescribed amount of chemical can be justified to assure the profitability of the crop. Therefore, the free market and economics do not protect you.

Yes, the food grown here in the Untied States still carries the risk of pesticide contamination. But there is more to the story. Over the years Americans have been growing accustomed to eating fruits and vegetables that are out of season in their own agricultural area. Perhaps they don't even grow in our country with the exception of some areas in Florida and southern California.

Bananas were the first to break the climate barrier nearly 50 years ago. United Fruit figured that one out and built an empire on it. Pineapple was next. The Hawaiian agricultural market, dominated by Dole, marketed the fruit, and bingo, pineapple was available practically all year long. Southern California and Florida developed a citrus industry that added more exotic fruit to the American diet. But that was not enough. Before long consumers wanted produce that perhaps grew locally, but only in season. They wanted strawberries and peaches in December. Freezing sort of worked for a while. By the 80's, not only did the vitamin industry become a mega-business, but also "fresh everything" became a requirement.

Everyone wanted fresh apples, peaches, pears, nectarines, mangoes, papayas, kiwi fruit, pineapples, melons, tomatoes, broccoli, and half a dozen forms of lettuce. You name it and consumers demanded it. No one seemed to care where or how it was grown, what chemicals covered it, or what bacteria; viruses and organisms were imbedded in it. After all, the government was there and the market economy would want to assure only healthy, happy consumers eating healthful, uncontaminated food.

Of course, the produce department in the local grocery store sprayed everything with a mist of water with regularity, giving the appearance of a fresh spring rain and a bountiful harvest. This did not hurt any illusions the marketing people were endeavoring to project. Apples, oranges and other produce were not left out of the show. Many of these received a fine wax coating (thereby protecting and sealing in whatever bad stuff was present) before they leave the food-processing center bound for local and long distance markets.

Meanwhile, inside cargo containers aboard ships for several days or weeks, cruising their way toward American consumer markets, new scientific technologies were being applied. This technology gives producers intriguing mixtures of gasses to use on food as it makes its way from Indonesia, Australia, Peru, Chile and Columbia to name but a few.

It is the *fresh look* that is so crucial. The grocer of today, as with the plastic surgeons that have sprung up like dandelions, are both attempting to create that *fresh look*. And the general public is eating it up. Pardon the pun.

With the appearance of this cornucopia of food, particularly the *fresh* produce, there are huge health risks that arise. However, these risks are not limited to the produce department. The deli, the seafood, the meat and poultry departments all threaten or can threaten you and your family.

For decades most people had only thought of food poisoning as good old ptomaine poisoning, which was normally limited to summer activities such as picnics, socials and potlucks. The big concern was to keep anything with mayonnaise cold since it was the rancidity of these heavy oil products, along with the potentially salmonella contaminated raw eggs, that was the culprit. Tuna, egg and chicken salads were very often guilty, especially if the sandwiches had been allowed to become warm. Thus the problem was more apparent at factories and job sites where lunch wagons were likely to sell food. Eating this food could be a fearful and uncomfortable event. Because communication was not what it is today, and life went on, as did the picnics, socials and potlucks. You just never heard much about people dying at a picnic as a result of eating a particular food. Rancid and putrid foodstuffs were occasionally encountered and our eyes and noses did a fine job of detecting these. The other warning was the bulging can. This was a dead giveaway of a problem. In the same manner, we avoided dented cans, especially if the contents were acidic as with tomatoes.

Local produce came to the market from local farmers, who could not afford to waste money on herbicides. They used hoes to take care of the weeds. Fungicides were not necessary since the plants were growing in basically healthy soils. When needed, water was used sparingly for irrigation. Some so-called insecticides, such as limewater, were used occasionally, but the bird, bat and snake populations were usually able to handle the bugs. Plants were planted in their season and harvested when ripe. The general theory at that time was to rinse the dirt off and you were ready to prepare dinner knowing that what you were preparing was healthy and healthful.

However, it is here that the problem fertilizers (i.e. manure) contaminated with E-Coli and salmonella were also being applied. To this day this fertilizer is still in those same "organic" fields, blowing around and being carried by the air and settling in the leaves of lettuce, cabbage and other layered vegetables, along with cucumbers and apples that are then waxed. This waxing preserves many types of bacteria and viruses.

Consider washing the outside of a head of lettuce and feeling secure that you have done your job. Now, take that same head of lettuce and using food coloring, soak the head of lettuce for a short period of time. Remove the head of lettuce from the water and pull it apart. This will reveal where the water has carried the coloring. You see, while this head of lettuce was growing and the leaves were being formed and layered, the airborne bacterium attached itself to and became entwined in the lettuce leaves. When this head of lettuce was harvested, it was possibly rinsed in water with all good intentions. However, rinsing the outside of this head of lettuce simply does not rid the lettuce of the airborne bacterium. Until now, the only way you could possibly address this problem would be to pull apart the head of lettuce and scrub each leaf separately, on both sides.

It's bad enough to live under the assumption that you can wash your produce well enough to remove pesticides used by American farming. But now with much of the produce coming from countries without any pesticide controls, your job is much more critical because what has penetrated the surface is basically nearly impossible for anyone to handle.

As the plant grew and developed its fruit, what it ingested is even more of a red flag. We have all read about or watched TV news about the problems in Mexico. The water irrigation supply used to water crops was pumped from a ditch that also serves as an open sewer. If the produce comes from Mexico, or other Latin American and Asian countries, then your produce may carry many surprising organisms as well as chemicals and heavy metals. Remember that water is the major constituent of most fruits and vegetables. Contaminated water will not only move *into* the plant's system, it will be deposited in its reproductive system. What we eat of the fruit or vegetable is really the plant's reproductive system.

Many may consider this information as hysterical ranting. No. It is serious and should be considered and discussed by more Americans. In the process of bringing more produce from other countries that have no real controls, rules or laws concerning chemicals or sanitation, there are people who, being aware of the conditions under which produce is grown and harvested, are refusing to buy this produce. The greed of the American free market entrepreneur is a powerful tool. So, now you will see produce boxes emblazoned with red, white & blue. The colors are printed in a ribbon style to give the illusion of an American flag. The box will then proudly state that the product was grown for and distributed BY xyz Company, located in Nowhere, Arizona. You will need reading glasses for the small print, but to a shopper it would appear that the tomatoes were grown right here in the USA.

Nonetheless, it is this subterfuge that these businesses are using. You see, you cannot print an American flag on the box because to have that symbol on the box means the produce had better be grown or produced here. But with a little imagination you are led to believe the produce is U.S. grown simply because of the red, white and blue artwork.

Just what kind of threats can these factors pose to you and your family?

Americans are definitely eating more fruits and vegetables. Much of this produce is being imported from countries with little or no control on what is used in the process, how this produce is handled when harvested in the field and on to the table. The responsibility to protect yourself and your family lies with you, the consumer.

In view of the conditions we are facing, what factors must you take into consideration before you allow yourself or your family to consume these products?

Early on we learned to rinse produce to remove dirt, pesticides and chemicals that may be present. No one ever mentioned a greater threat, one that rinsing, or washing will not eliminate.

We know that bacteria and other organisms are present on all of our fruits and vegetables. But, has anyone considered the fact that some of those organisms may have been present when chemicals and pesticides were applied, or that some of them may have survived to become much more virulent? Perhaps they mutated and now have the ability to inflict a different kind of damage as a result of various chemical encounters. Assuredly, rinsing the vegetable or fruit in water is not quite going to do the job. Neither is the rinsing done by food processors. It is these very undeniable facts that will increasingly make the news headlines in the near future.

These potential threats come from fruits and vegetables that are notorious for high pesticide levels such as apples, grapes, green beans, peaches, pears, spinach and winter squash. However, the threat posed by those that are generally lower in pesticide residue, such as bananas, broccoli, canned peaches, corn and frozen or canned peas, is just as real, if not worse. The organisms on these fruits and vegetables can develop into more numerous and sturdier organisms with greater potential immunity. The crucial fact is that the very things we must consume for a healthy life are now potentially detrimental to our health.

THE POISONS OF PROTEIN

We are now to the point where bacteria like salmonella and E-Coli can be found even on sprouts. In the past, salmonella was hardly ever encountered. Only recently we have come to know about salmonella, and its effects, mainly with poultry and eggs. The poultry, pork and beef industries of this country have always been an area of primary concern for the federal and state departments of agriculture, followed by the dairy industry. Even fish was never given much notice by these enforcers of food safety.

Despite the focus of the inspection systems, the holes are getting bigger. More and more threats are going to face us at the market. Having mentioned salmonella earlier, in June 1999, salmonella was discovered in non-pasteurized orange juice, hardly a meat or poultry product. So even our preconceived notions of what can be infected with what are no longer valid.

The two most notorious bacteria on the street, because they are so very lethal, are E-Coli and Listeria. Finding its way into products such as hot dogs and lunchmeat, Listeria killed 11 people in 1999. Thorn Apple Valley had produced 30,000,000 lbs. (or 15,000 tons) of these toxic hot dogs at their Forrest City, Arkansas factory. Oscar Meyer recalled 10.8 tons of deli meats that were infected with Listeria. Tyson Foods of Arkansas recalled about 78,000 chicken burritos for Listeria infection. Sara Lee, a subsidiary of BilMar Foods of Michigan, producers of hot dogs and deli meats, recalled its production after 17 died and 65 were sickened. Milk products produced by Kohler Mix Specialties of Minnesota, did not escape the Listeria bacteria. B & B Meat & Sausage of Washington recalled 1500 lbs. of their Hempler brand franks and knockwurst. No fatalities.

It is very frightening to realize that the meat and poultry products found to be infected were not raw products. These were finished, cooked, packaged and ready to go on a picnic or for your sandwich at lunch. How could anyone have suspected a problem? We are talking about BallPark Franks, Oscar Meyer Deli Meats and Tyson's Chicken Burritos, which are often served as airline meals.

Listeria had been out of the news since 1985 when Jalisco's brand of soft cheese, (not meat or poultry) sickened 142 people and killed 40. It has shown its ugly head again. Is this the harbinger of things to come? To many concerned medical professionals it is. To those who have been affected by any of these potentially fatal threats, tomorrow has arrived today.

E-Coli, once considered to be easily kept at bay by good sanitary practices on the part of anyone involved in food handling, is now more rampant than ever before. Many organisms learned long before we humans showed up with our bactericides, germicides and antibiotics, that change and adaptation is the basis of survival. E-Coli was not to be caught unprepared. Now we face a version of this old bacterium, E-Coli 0157:H7. This new mutation is tough and current antibiotics are no match for it.

Whether this new form of E-Coli developed in reaction to antibiotic overuse, or came from some infectious disease hotspot such as Southeast Asia, South and Central America, or the train station in New Delhi, we do not know. We do know we have encountered it, named it and now must be alert for it while taking steps to keep it out of the food supply system.

93

This new mutation of E-Coli was actually first encountered in the early 80's. In 1993, at the Jack in the Box chain, E-Coli was responsible for the death of 4 youngsters on the West Coast. In 1997, it struck Hudson Foods and Beef of America.

Though normally transmitted through beef, particularly hamburger or ground beef, in 1996 nearly 9,000 Japanese were infected. E-Coli was traced to radish sprouts of all things! Here at home, in 1999, a 16-month-old toddler died and 65 people were sickened after drinking infected apple juice produced by the Odwalla Company.

So, what is a person to do? If what you read in magazines or newspapers, hear on the radio or television gives you pause for concern, it should. With the growth of the world's population, those good old American icons of food processing will be doing their production on a worldwide basis. The flow of produce from countries such as Mexico, with its aversion to high sanitation standards and chemical regulation usage, has provided us with a basic sketch of the future.

The solution will not lie with the medical community. Do not look to the government. The lobbying power of the international agribusiness is growing and their big customers, (McDonald's, Burger King, Jack in the Box and so on) will not interfere with the flow of cheap supplies. Those cheap supplies assure them of ever-greater profits. Many doing the work at processing plants here in this country are not locals. They are imported labor from places where the most basic concepts of sanitation have never existed. For example, the town of Huntingberg, Indiana, an old German farming community in southern Indiana with an unemployment rate of 1 or 2%, is going to be the home of a huge turkey processing plant. Who will be employed? Not the locals. Hundreds of imported cheap labor Mexicans and Central Americans, who are inexperienced with sanitary processing methods, will fill these jobs.

The threat of tainted food is at every level; from the market to the cafeteria, the restaurant, the fast food outlet, the finest hotels and resorts. All pose the same threat to us when we consume anything coming through the food supply system. The infection may come from the field, from the irrigation water, from the harvesters, from the truckers, from the delivery persons, or the produce employees, cooks, kitchen help, servers and even you. All of these can introduce the organisms individually or as an entire chain of persons, each contributing along the way. As you can see, the introduction of a growing number of lethal bacteria and viruses is growing, by leaps and bounds.

Some still believe that the infections resulting from eating poisonous or contaminated food shouldn't be of that much concern to us because modern medical technology always comes to the rescue. This is a positive faith in the men and women who do use every available resource to solve problems. However, even they are getting concerned about the power of their weapons against a flexible and ever-changing enemy.

CHAPTER 5

THE BATTLE OF THE BIOLOGICALS VS. OUR FAMILIES IS THERE A WAY TO WIN?

Why are so many antibiotics no longer able to do their jobs? Why do we have to use newer and stronger antibiotics? Several paths have led us to the crisis concerning the efficiency of antibiotics.

The oldest of these pathways originated in the 50's. It was during this time that consumers were first being ingrained with the knowledge and fear of germs. Germs were everywhere and if you somehow achieved a germ-free home, your worries were over. Gas stations and restaurants were promoting germ-free restrooms. This was achieved by mounting an ultra-violet light on the toilet. When the cover was lifted the light was supposed to turn off. Sometimes it did not. There were ultraviolet lights killing germs at medical offices, dental offices and who know where else. Motels touted sheets that were treated with ultraviolet. However, ultraviolet lights were not very practical in the home. Enter the germ killers in a bottle.

Lysol was the answer, or perhaps Pine Sol or some other concoction in a bottle that killed germs. At Halloween, unwrapped candy and any other yummy looking unwrapped goodies that might have been touched by germ-laden hands were immediately disposed of. Along came cellophane and new plastic wrap companies who fed the fuel of this paranoia. The hand soap manufacturers were very enthused about washing your hands a dozen times an hour. You could watch their profits soar as you watched the soap dissolve before your very eyes.

As with so many American activities, we went overboard. A lot of us became germ freaks. Before long even straws for everything from soda pop to milkshakes were wrapped. Incidentally, those wrappers were perfect for spitballs (which surely were a "direct shot" in delivering and spreading germs.) Not everyone got into the germ phobia. There were, then as now, a lot of people who are not big on germs or basic cleanliness. Nonetheless, they were affected by this germicidal tidal wave.

The problem with attempting to achieve germ-free, or seemingly super-clean conditions, is sort of like unilateral disarmament with a foe that does not care if he dies to kill you. We are at a real disadvantage. This is war; a war that we humans are losing more and more by the day. Put into an understandable perspective, think of a nuclear holocaust killing 40 million people. Unless we address the virus and bacteria problem the potential for catastrophe will make the nuclear annihilation pale in comparison.

Because so many of us grew up in a germ phobic environment, we were more susceptible to various kinds of infections and reactions that should not have affected us at all. Those of us born after WWII are too often just as easily bothered by minor kinds of reactions we should have been immune to. Lacking some of these immunities we should have gained during our early years, all too often we are deficient in the ability to fend off more complex and stronger forms of bacteria and virus now.

The germ phobia of the 50's and thereafter may have resulted in less self-immunities and natural immunities. However, another very potent factor was at work from, of all sources, our food supplies. It was most certainly the meat and poultry industries that did us the greatest harm in those days. Yes indeed, they should bear much of the blame for the failure of so many antibiotics to do their jobs today. By the late 50's and onward, the use of antibiotics in the beef, pork and poultry industries became absurd.

The feed given these animals was laced with the same antibiotics used on humans. Rather than be concerned with raising these animals in more sanitary conditions with less crowding, it was cheaper to feed animals inexpensive antibiotics. By the late 60's, it was common to give cattle, before being loaded onto trucks and rail cars, and shipped off to meat processors, an injection of streptomycin (a very large cow sized injection.) As the beef-on-the-hoof was herded on the truck or train after receiving their injection, they walked perhaps 50 feet. At the other end of the ride, they walked perhaps another 300 feet at most. The total time from injection to slaughter is a period of 12-20 hours.

As a result of this procedure, everyone eating any beef product has, at one time or another received a dose of streptomycin. Over enough time, and enough hamburgers, we eventually ended up with an antibiotic that was no longer able to function in its original intended capacity. It could not function because the very targets it was aimed at were all quite immune to it. This is the result of years of injections given to cows. The antibiotic was neutralized. 10,000 cattle in a feedlot represent *Big Money* and *BIG* disease potential. So, use antibiotics and who's going to lose?

However, this was not limited to beef. Pork and poultry also have had the same practices carried on for the same reason—money. It is cheaper to give animals antibiotics than to risk losing them to the real problems, mainly poor sanitation due to over-crowding.

In American capitalism, the effects of these kinds of decisions are never made with any concern except the long-term effects on today's bottom-line accounting decisions. Never have. Never will.

Is it any wonder that so many good, old antibiotics are worthless today? Yes, the organisms that attack us have been changing thus requiring newer and newer antibiotics. But what motivated these changes, these mutations? It was their instinct for survival in the face of antibiotics introduced into our bodies every time we ate meat or poultry. We owe all of this to our agribusiness systems and their profit margins.

So, with natural immunities reduced by the germicidal campaigns run by the soap industry, the antibiotics being compromised and virtually negated by our consumption, in low doses, of the same antibiotics when we ate, any immunity to fend off nearly anything was compromised to some extent. Unfortunately, now our children and grandchildren are suffering the consequences.

An entire new generation of children is facing a very new and to some extent dangerous set of circumstances that have arisen as a result of the previous practices described. Once again, this threat is the result of economics.

In today's society, parents have to work to make ends meet. For the single parent families the economics of today leaves them no choice. Everyday across America, children are rousted from their beds and hauled off to daycare centers and pre-schools. Some children are taken to private homes, some are taken to public facilities, and still others are taken to private facilities. All of these facilities have rules against admitting children who are exhibiting various levels of sickness. Yet 90% of the illness comes from the very daycare, preschool or private facilities the children occupy for 8—10 hours a day.

At the first sign of a sniffle the child is quickly whisked to the doctor for medication. As a result and in most cases, the majority of youngsters have received many antibiotics that they should not have received at all. When added to the previous antibiotic programs with beef, pork and poultry, we are beginning to see that our arsenal of antibiotics has become so compromised we now require even stronger antibiotics, and some simply do not work anymore. Thus, every day, each of us is more and more at risk of becoming seriously ill as a result of bacteria, viruses and germs that 50 years ago would not have affected us.

Not only are these germs more able to wreak havoc, they may be a more evolved or a mutant version with immunity to our antibiotic. In essence, our evolution has taken a step backward by making us more susceptible to more and more evolved germs.

This is why the foods we prepare and eat at home must be handled with caution and sanitation. It is also why eating out is an occasion that places us at risk.

Perhaps many of us will again be growing our vegetables in our own gardens. *A WORD OF CAUTION:* Use good, clean organic materials. Use peat moss, straw, vermiculite, perlite, ground bark and/or wood chips (nitrolized.) So-called composted recycled commercial products are not what they should be. *KEEP THE COMPOST VEGETARIAN.* Table scraps such as meat, fish or poultry will turn the compost into a rancid useless pile of maggots, rats and all sorts of bad stuff.

CHAPTER 6

CATCHING MORE THAN A FLIGHT IN THE FRIENDLY SKIES

In recent years, the new communication breakthroughs have not eliminated the need for business trips. As commerce becomes more international, so do those business trips. Additionally, an increasing number of families board airplanes for flights around the globe as well as flights to visit relatives. Add to this, the virtual tidal wave of cruise ships plying the seas for days or weeks, most loaded with not just a few hundred but with upwards to thousands or more people. With these thoughts in mind we realize just how often and how readily that we can encounter threats to our health never before conceived.

Take a moment and consider the international flight you are boarding to return home. That jet has been flying from airport to airport, loading and unloading people and baggage. No matter where you are, the locals clean your plane, they prepare your food, but they do not clean the air filters or duct work nor do they replace the carbon filters which allegedly purify the air you will be breathing for the next 4, 6, 8 or more hours. Except for a few cities in the world (if that many) the locals haven't a hint of what clean is, much less any other concept of sanitation. Did they wash their hands before making that sandwich you will be eating?

Numerous backsides from anywhere and everywhere have occupied the seats. Clothing that was dirty. The pants of the last man sitting in your seat may have been on the floor of the Men's Room at the Bombay Train Station, or on the floor of the airport in Nigeria. Now you are sitting in that seat, and when you get home your 5-year-old is going to be happily tugging the seat of your pants wanting to be picked up. The airplane's carpet harbors what shoes have walked on; urine wetted floors, toilet overflows containing fecal matter, and you want to slip your shoes off to rest your feet on the carpet!

How about overhead? See those little stained vents? It's been years since any cigarette smoke has been there, so what is it? It's dirt and every sort of bacteria gathered from the air and sucked into those vents mixed with the little critters expelled by coughs and sneezes. Some of those coughs and sneezes may have had tuberculosis or any of a dozen other aliments that are transmitted in the air. Over the next 2, 4, 6, 8 hours or more you and all of your fellow passengers will be adding to that mix. Moisture will also be added at the rate of one quart per hour. This moisture will be in the form of perspiration and respiration. On a 4 hour flight with just 100 people on board a total of 100 gallons of water mixed with all of these various organisms is made available for everyone to breathe. A few may find a resting-place on your person or your clothes in their effort to survive and the chance to reproduce. But those few are all that are needed.

Add to that already stuffy, dirty mess in the air of the jet plane is the new decision to change the air circulation in the cabin from 15 cubic feet a minute to 5 cubic feet a minute. In short, now you will literally breathe the same dirty, germ-laden air 3 times longer. To put this into perspective, a large garbage bag holds about 32 gallons or 4 cubic feet. Until now the airlines allowed you to have almost 4 trash bags of so-called filtered air every minute. Now the plan is to give you only 1 trash bag of "more concentrated" filtered air per minute. There is definitely a difference between 4 trash bags of so-called filtered air and 1 trash bag of "more concentrated" filtered air. Air travel that results in colds, cold symptoms, nasal congestion, headaches or tiredness for you or members of your family today will only get worse.

Flatulence on the plane, with this new air change policy will not allow for dissipation of the gaseous releases as readily as before. Using the overhead air blower may assist you. However, at this new rate of air exchange we may literally have an odorous haze all around us!

The Love Boat brought the idea of cruising back. However, it did not bring American flagships with American crews. Foreign crews are serving most cruise ships. As long as cruise lines charge enough and want repeat business, the quality will be there. However, there are a number of lesser quality cruise ships who, although charging high prices, do not provide ideal sanitary bathroom conditions, air quality control, and quality control of the kitchen and its migrant workers is questionable, along with food service control. Because of the close quarters, the Tropical zones these ships ply, and the lack of quality control food storage, handling and inspection, a pleasure cruise may be a catastrophic incident waiting to happen not only for a food borne bug but also airborne organisms through unclean and non-inspected ventilation systems.

The point here is that with today's modern technology and sanitary techniques available there is no reason not to assure anyone anywhere of safe and healthy access to quality controlled clean air, sanitary facilities, along with food processing, storage, handling, preparing and serving in a clean environment. The only reason for not employing these techniques is the ugly head of economics. If the air ductwork of the ships is kept clean, the odds for contamination are somewhat reduced.

The advent of cheap labor, year-round production, over-use or misuse of pesticides, foul air in air planes and the conditions existing on cruise ships has the effect of placing anyone who travels and, in turn, all of us in jeopardy at any given time.

How can we protect our families and ourselves? Is there a technology already in place to successfully deal with these most complex yet basic problems? The answer is a resounding YES! Not only can the health and well being of your family and yourself be assured, you can also help others achieve these goals to your benefit financially as well as healthfully.

CHAPTER 7

FOCUSING ON OUR HOMES

To this point our focus has been the identification of the myriad sources of dangers that confront you and your family. From the materials used to construct or remodel your home, the materials that go into the painting and carpeting, along with new furnishings you replace, to the dangers from the well insulated, energy efficient home designs being marketed nationwide.

We also touched on the so-called global market and how you are the helpless consumer purchasing what you believe to be healthy food. You don't know where the food has been grown, in what conditions or how the food was handled. You have come to realize that these dangers are to be found everywhere, from the local fast food restaurant, to the upscale eateries, to your own home.

For those in the fast lane of commerce and business, you have become aware of the health dangers from jet travel and how even your vacations can endanger your health. However, warnings and fear do not solve the problems. The home, the food, the vacation are all part of life and no one is going into a corner and hide. And if you did, who knows what dangers lurk in the corner?

Therefore, the reasonable answer is to take reasonable actions to reduce the potential dangers while enjoying your home, your dining either at home or out, when you travel or when you do all the other things that we humans enjoy doing. Life is a risk; we all take risks every day. It's called living and it involves using our reason, our intelligence, knowledge and experience that make those risks acceptable. Our mind and its information retrieval systems are constantly at work reducing every day risks to acceptable levels. This same reasonable thinking provides us with a relatively safe day and can be brought into play when it comes to the dangers we have previously discussed.

IDENTIFYING & LOCATING SOURCES OF POSSIBLE CONTAMINATIONS

THE NOSE KNOWS! That wonderfully amazing sensor, the nose, alerts us to the good, bad, or dangerous toxic odors all around us. If there is an odd odor that causes a bell to sound in your mind, you had better heed the warning. The nose knows! There is an old saying in the real estate business; "smell does not sell"

Generally, people ignore and do not link a musty, irritating odor or other noticeable bad odor(s) to a sick home. Many people choose to ignore odors that are caused by living and dying viruses and bacteria, caused by so-called *simple molds*. Molds are not simple (it's just a musty smell), but they are, in fact, the underlying cause of many illnesses and in many cases, can prove to be deadly.

These so-called *simple molds* have names such as *pennicillium, aspergillus* and *cladosporium*. These white-green, blue-green and dark brown fungi can grow anywhere. Even *stachybotrys atra*, which may produce poisons that cause internal bleeding, has been found growing in the interior of homes and buildings.

Always remember; if there is even a trace of a bad, foul smell, the nose is giving you an advanced warning of a huge potential problem. The choice is yours. Take heed of the warning, or ignore it and suffer the consequences.

So, what is a sick home? What causes the sick home syndrome?

The cold hard facts are an entire spectrum of noticeable indicators that can point toward the culprit that is the cause of endless, identified and unidentified reasons for illnesses related to the home environment.

If someone in your home has any symptoms ranging from a constant, stuffy, runny nose, coughing, fatigue, inability to concentrate, always tired, nausea, sneezing, headaches, red, itchy, runny eye irritations, ignoring the signs and sweeping things under the rug, (no pun intended) is not going to help or make the environment better. Unless dealt with, the problem will grow and become worse and worse.

If there is a musty odor, a stench, or stinky bad smells as if something is rotting or dying, that's a tip off to a very serious problem. *THE NOSE KNOWS!* Yet sometimes the sick home syndrome conditions can be caused by conditions that escape even the most sensitive nose. These can be degassing vapors from man-made materials used in construction and furnishings.

Ferreting out or isolating the source of the problem can sometimes be an impossible task. If that becomes the case, the only recourse is the good old "shotgun" treatment approach. Perhaps you have isolated some of the problem. Nevertheless, a full-scale treatment that covers the entire home is a definite must. What you know, see, and have found is one thing; but the unseen, the unfound and the unknown will also get caught up in the treatment, and in the process, will also be eliminated.

Blunt talk from *The Nose* needs no apology. If the symptoms are present, let the reader judge the risks.

Let's start at the front door. Entry can be very revealing for smells and odors. As stated earlier in this book, what is offensive or irritating to one person may be part of another person's environment, even if it's detrimental. People living within certain environments become accustomed to the atmosphere around them, and may even have become conditioned to the elements that surround them. This can lead to a blissful unawareness on their part, but certainly not on our part.

More often than not, smells and odors are an indicator that the place could stand a good airing out and are always a dead give away of nasty problems.

During the process of living, breeding and dying, molds, mildews and other bacteria and viruses produce toxic spores that float all over in the air within the house causing a toxic soup that used to be known as *stale air.*

Okay, what do you say we take a walk through the house? As we step through the door into the entryway, we are now in the environment of the habitat.

> • Was there a catchall debris mat before we came in the door to trap at least some of the nasties on our shoes?

> • Is there a rug inside the door to help contain the nasties on our shoes so at least some of that bad stuff stays on that rug?

We continue into the living room.

At one time or another everyone has sat in a living room and gazed into a ray of sunshine visible within the room, and has seen a lot of what they thought were minute dust particles just floating in the air. All of those particles consist of numerous uncounted and unidentified spores, pollens, chemical gases, smoke, molecules, animal dander, animal urine/feces residue, dust mite feces, germs, and bacteria that our bodies are exposed to, and have to deal with. Those very particles floating around may be known as illness-causing allergens.

It always reminds us of the housekeeper whose main tool was a good old feather duster. In the process of "dusting," the housekeeper was constantly stirring up and whipping around all of the above nasty ingredients known as "dust" while commenting, "every time I do this it makes me sneeze a lot and causes me to get terrible headaches."

The activity of dusting, or more properly stated, scattering, "*I'll just whip it around a little here, a little there and I'll have this place ship shape in no time at all*," is really, "*I'll have it all floating and scattered in the air again until it settles, then I'll paddle it around and around again and again and again*," instead of dealing with it once and for all by vacuuming it up with a good efficient vacuum system.

The simple fact is, it's better to leave it (the dust) lay where it is and even build up to a layer, than it is to swish it around into the air that we breath. So you see, those cute little "Dust Bunnies" aren't so cute after all.

- Are there pets?

- Are there atmospheric residue producing plants that for some people can be a problem, unbeknownst to them?

- Are there over-whelming smells from potpourri and other so-called air fresheners (chemical cover ups only) or perfumes that can do more harm than good?

- Are there musty smells, smoker's residue, and new furniture or carpet smells that are, in fact, degassing odors?

• Along with all that spare change, what else is in between those couch cushions?

Any and all of these things can contribute to the cause of a *Sick Unhealthy Home*. The trick is to isolate the problems, and then to deal with them.

Now let's move on over to the kitchen and get right down to business. Let's pull that refrigerator out and take a look. Wow! Look at all the dust, dirt, and lint! "Hey, I was wondering where those keys went." Then we look on top of the fridge and the cupboards. Well, hello Dust Bunnies!

Now take a look under the sink that is right next to the dishwasher. The dishwasher is doing its thing, going through its normal cycle. We feel the hot, moist air that the dishwasher is feeding into the cabinet under the sink, to say nothing about a small water leak or spillage. This is definitely a breeding ground for lots of germs, mold, mildew, bacteria, viruses, and all kinds of other nasty life forms.

Kitchens are where we deposit the groceries we bring home along with all of those endless potential nasties that were created in the process of producing and people handling. Ever think about that?

Preparation is very critical; cleanliness, in this case, is Godliness. Otherwise it could very well be detrimental to our well-being, health and happiness.

Let's not forget those long dark mazes known as hallways that everyone tends to overlook. Don't forget, pets also use these thoroughfares. Plus, they are pathways for any other bugs or inhabitants that are present that you may or may not be aware of or acquainted with. All of these combine to distribute everything from dander to feces. The rule doesn't change— take extra care to vacuum them and their residue up, and toss them out.

Bathrooms, the nursery for major breeding areas of every imaginable known and unknown germ, such as mold spores, fungi, viruses, and bacteria. Damp and moist areas are perfect for such activity. Try to keep these areas dry with lots of fresh air circulating. Check it out; every nook and cranny of the bathroom is subject to the suspicion of donating harmful stuff:

- Loose caulking around showers and tubs,

- Water collecting and left standing,

- Very minor, inconsequential leaks that can grow into monstrous problems such as dry rot, (which is *very expensive to correct,*) not to mention that it's also very unhealthy.

Recreation (wreck room) or family room; this is the room that the whole family usually spends most of their time in. We eat, drink sleep, relax, watch TV, have parties, play games, and entertain in this room.

For whom is this a recreation room? Think of all the human and or pet food residues that collect under furniture. This is a virtual smorgasbord for cockroaches and our little buddy, "the Dust Mite." Don't forget the damp areas due to spillage and possible pet urine. Yes, this is real recreation, for all the other inhabitants too, not just humans.

Ahh, the bedroom; that cozy, safe area where we sleep, rest and get away from the world. It's where we spend almost half of our lifetime. And while we are sleeping, resting and getting away from the world, we are not alone. Guess who's awake. That's right, our little lifelong companions, the "Dust Mites" and uncounted other critters too numerous to mention. They are eating, breeding, living and dying, just like us *except* they are smaller, a whole lot smaller. They get their rest and sleep when we are not around. When we show up in that bed, it's party time and chow time!

Sure, we can spare that shedding skin they feed on, except for one thing. In the process of eating our flakes of skin, they (the Dust Mites) turn that very meal into deadly feces. Then we, in turn, breathe it into our lungs, it gets in our eyes and nose making them itch, and consequently, very bad things happen. This was again reaffirmed in an article of the Seattle Times dated Tuesday, January 20, 2000. Not only was the Dust Mite issue addressed, but also all of the other inhabitants sharing our cozy little bedrooms with us as well.

Lauran Neergaard, of The Associated Press, wrote the article appearing in the Seattle Times, it reads as follows:

> WASHINGTON: As doctors struggle to understand why asthma is rising at an alarming rate, a new report concludes that microscopic dust mites lurking in carpets and bedding can push children who are susceptible to asthma, but don't yet have it, to develop the disease.
>
> About 17.3 million Americans have asthma, a respiratory disease that leaves sufferers coughing, wheezing, and gasping for air. Cases of asthma have risen about 75 percent since 1980, particularly among blacks and poor, inner-city populations, says the report released yesterday by the Institute of Medicine.
>
> Doctors have long warned that certain allergens can worsen patients' asthma, triggering or exacerbating attacks of breathlessness. But no one can explain why new cases are rising so dramatically. "This is a major problem," said Dr. Richard Johnston of the University of Colorado, who chaired the Institute of Medicine committee. "There are genes that affect your susceptibility to asthma, but the genes could not have changed over that period of time," he said. "Something else has changed. It means something in the environment."

His committee didn't solve that mystery, but the new report may serve as a practical guide to what in the indoor environment affects asthma, and what practical steps could ease symptoms.

The conclusion: Dust mites, cockroaches, cat dander and, for preschool children, breathing second-hand tobacco smoke are some of the proven culprits in making asthma worse. The mere existence of dust mites may not be the sole cause of a person's asthma, because mites live in nearly all homes. But in children genetically susceptible to asthma, exposure to dust mites can lead to the disease, the report says.

The report offers simple strategies to ease asthmatics' symptoms:

- Encase mattresses and pillows in plastic covers, opt for leather sofas instead of upholstery, and get rid of carpets, all favorite hideouts for dust mites
- Never allow smoking inside the house.
- Remove pets and then thoroughly clean to remove their dander.
- Exterminate cockroaches.
- Control indoor humidity, because dust mites particularly, and also cockroaches, thrive in humid conditions.

The article pretty much says it all, except that there is a major breakthrough to help us to deal with this oh, so serious problem. (The SCO Technologies, Inc certified Medallion Healthy Homes System.)

Let's not overlook or forget another habitat we maintain for our little guests, be they rodents, insects, or arachnids. Dark, enclosed closets and storage places are the perfect place, quiet and undisturbed. You can't get it any better if you're one of these little guests.

What goes on in there is another world, but it can affect your whole life. You store the things you use there, what you wear, your bedding, towels, shoes and so on. Every time you open and close that door, you are contributing to those nasty little critters' well being. And at the same time,

9-OCON

contributing, by fanning into the air in the rooms where those closets are located, all those deadly spores, viruses, and feces that can cause illnesses for many people.

Many times we have all heard the old saying, "so and so keeps a good, clean house, it's so clean you can eat off the floor." For our little guests in our homes, this could very well be a true statement, possibly a real banquet!

The menu could read as this:

- Appetizers anyone? For openers, we have cat dander with breadcrumbs, or dog hair with grass, freshly dragged in from the yard, with just a hint of lemon floor cleaner.

- Drinks anyone? Our open bar offers well drinks such as standing water next to the toilet, or for the connoisseur of fine liquids, we have, aged in wood, under the sink waters, gently blended with all of the many cleaning compounds and cleaners. An assortment of vintages that will titillate even the most discriminating pallet!

- The soup of the day is: Hair Follicle DeJour, or Cream of Lint.

- The main entrée is absolutely the largest collection and a variety of edibles in nature! The mixes and matches in our banquet are endless, which of course, will be eaten off the floor.

- We begin with lemon flavored floor wax and move on to numerous other chemicals/cleaners to clean your palate.

- Then, feel free to help yourself to our skin flake salad bar. Ladies and gentlemen, friends and strangers, acquaintances and unknowns, don't be shy! Step right up and help yourselves!

- For dessert, we have animal droppings, and for after dinner drinks, we have especially aged (warm or cold) cat and dog urine.

No, we cannot create a risk-free environment, but with some reason, and informative intelligent facts plus our own knowledge and experience, we can achieve a safer environment for our families and ourselves.

H.E.P.A.
(HIGH EFFICIENCY PARTICULATE ARRESTORS)

Over the past several years we have heard more and more about a filter known as a HEPA filter. Originally, these filters were designed to filter air being circulated in CLEAN ROOMS. These are rooms used to manufacture silicon chips or semi-conductors. They are kept virtually contaminant free through the use of large-scale ionizers and filters (HEPA filters.) HEPA filters were quite costly after their introduction; however, today they are quite reasonable and should be used in the home.

On the other hand, do not be misled by the marketing of so-called *room air purifiers*. These appliances are sold nearly everywhere but do they work as they are supposed to? By and large, these appliances use a fan, a rudimentary electrostatic grid or ionizer and, of course, a HEPA filter. The most commonly marketed room air purifier costs about $149.00 and claims to have the ability to clean the air in a 16' x 20' room six times per hour. In addition, with its HEPA filter it can *delete* 99.97% of all airborne contaminants such as allergens and other particles. Sounds too good to be true, and it is.

At first thought, one assumes that a 16' x 20' room with 8' ceilings encompassing 2560 cubic feet will, with a 300 cubic foot per minute fan should be able to literally make the room 99% pure in 8 to 10 minutes. That is what the advertising would lead you to believe. But now, as Paul Harvey says, "the rest of the story."

If the 16' x 20' room has no corners and no windows, and the wall, ceiling and floor surfaces are slick and static free, and we suspend such a unit in the center of the room half way between the floor and the ceiling, we might actually clean up some air. But how much?

First of all, we can't forget the air currents created when we turn this appliance on. In one minute it will have processed 300 cubic feet of air. However, the 300 cubic feet of processed air within the immediate proximity (a diameter circle of approximately 5 or 6 feet) will not displace another 300 cubic feet. It will mix with the existing processed air in that same area and the same air will go through the system again and again and again. Each minute 300 cubic feet of air is moved through the appliance, but the percentage of untreated air remaining to be processed will not reduce as fast as one might think.

The actual flow should be measured in seconds. A 300 CFM (cubic feet per minute) fan will push about 5 cubic feet per second through the unit on the next trip through. These 5 cubic feet may pick up in its currents an additional 5% of unprocessed air, or about .25 cubic feet per second. From that point on the amount of unprocessed air brought through will fall as the mixing process becomes less and less active as we move away from the unit.

So, the 300 CFM capacity of the fan has no real relationship to the amount of air processed or purified simply because of the mixing effect. In reality, there are at best 15 cubic feet of, 99% pure air in the first minute. After an hour, the amount being purified drops, as air further away from the machine does not get processed. In about 10 days, running 24 hours per day, this room would probably approach the 90% + mark in its immediate vicinity (that same 5 or 6 foot circle.)

Now using the same appliance in a normal room, with windows, furnishings, carpets, shelves and so on, you would need at least 8 machines mounted halfway up each wall and several spaced around the room. Providing the room is not opened for 10 to 20 days you may have some fairly pure air. However, the feces of dust mites, dander, spores and other biologicals that remain undisturbed will not be eliminated because they have not been stirred up. If anything, they will benefit from pure, uncontaminated air, to say nothing of the dank musty smell that will result in the mix of pure air and home humidity.

In so many words, these devices are nearly worthless in any living space where adults, children and their pets live and play and doors open and close, and people come and go. In so many words, these devices are really a waste of money and do little, if anything to help make your home healthy.

A home should stop being a sealed living container with you and your family members rebreathing the same old air loaded with contaminants that are created and flourish in this type of environment. Doesn't it make sense to create a healthy home where your children come and go, friends visit and doors open and close and you and your family can enjoy life without everyone living as though they are in a space ship, and a poorly designed one at that?

I remember the farmhouse I was raised in and the homes I have lived in since. Sure, the fresh air of the outdoors came in through spaces around the windows and doors and from any little crack that let it in. These homes changed the air frequently. Sure, it took a little more heat in the winter and a little more air conditioning in the summer, but it was worth it. And you know what? It is far cheaper to use a little more gas or electricity than it is to pay for the doctor's visits, prescriptions and a much less healthy life for both you and your family.

As a matter of fact, after you have undone the damage done to you, your family and your home by having the Medallion Healthy Home treatment, you should finally let the fresh air in. Open the windows just a crack (1/8"), put a higher CFM fan in the bathrooms and vent it outdoors. You might consider having the air feeding your heater and air conditioning come from outside, through a regularly changed HEPA filter, and your home will get healthy as well as your family.

To carry this a step further, have 2 small exhaust fans of say, 100 CFM installed on the outer walls of each room. One should be placed about 2 ft. from the floor and the other 2 ft. from the ceiling. Again, on an outside wall and opposite or diagonal from the vents that deliver heated or cooled air.

To make this exhaust system smart, wire the fan closest to the ceiling to operate when the air conditioner is operating. For the fan closest to the floor wire it to operate when the heat system is in operation. As a result, when you are heating the house, this cooler more dense air falls and it and its cargo of odors, dander, spores and so on are dumped outdoors. Likewise, in the summer when you are cooling the house, the warmer, lighter air will rise and be vented outside with its cargo of the same biological and chemical pollution will be removed from you home.

Perhaps you are worried about efficiency and expense. Right now your *energy* efficient home is really only causing short and long-term health problems, and even more so for your children.

Using this technology you will probably see no added cost for energy and big savings in health costs. Remember, you are bringing outdoor air, filtered by a HEPA type filter into the system. As the air approaches the heating space in your furnace it will already be gaining heat as it enters. The same is true for fresh filtered air coming into the cooling grid of the air conditioner. No, you are not going to see much, if any, energy cost increase. You will see an increase in vitality and well being of those for whom the house is a home.

CHAPTER 8

A NATURAL WAY TO FIGHT THE CHEMICAL & BIOLOGICAL WARS IN OUR HOMES

When I thought about writing this book, I knew that I had to convince an entire nation of people who, for several generations, have been brainwashed and misled into believing false ideas about ozone. The fact that ozone is Nature's oxidizer has been demonstrated, confirmed and reconfirmed over and over. Ozone can effectively destroy most known bacteria and viruses. There simply is not one scintilla of published data to refute this statement.

The unchallenged dogma left the uninformed public not only misinformed but also misdirected. No one was ever told that ozone (by itself) could kill life threatening viruses, germs and bacteria such as *E-Coli, hepatitis, salmonella, and streptococcus.*

Very seldom do the purported experts reverse their supposed expert mindset. That mindset occurred by way of their incomplete search for knowledge and information regarding ozone. After all, a lifetime of beliefs is just that, a lifetime of beliefs be they right or wrong. It is nearly impossible to admit that all of your work has been on the wrong track, especially if you laid down the track. Being committed to your beliefs, even when all other evidence is overwhelmingly against you, is not only catastrophic for you, but most of all detrimental for millions of your fellow human beings who rely on your purported (but very questionable) expertise.

What would happen if millions of people learned, by word of mouth, that the information about ozone that was force-fed to them was only one part of the story? As Paul Harvey was very fond of saying, "now for the rest of the story." That has never been truer than in the writing of this "other side of the story."

There are many people throughout the world and in the United States, within the scientific community, who were aware of the revealing untruths, half truths and misinformation, yet are unwilling to face up to their responsibilities because of the possible damaging personal ramification. "Best left unsaid, then I don't have to deal with it" syndrome. I admit that attempting to explain this phenomenon without using words such as *intellectually dishonest* is tough. However, for these people and the media fear of ozone-laden smog sells better that fresh air.

This serious accusation is not made from arrogance, but rather with deep concern that the errors of the rest of the world are so wide spread as to threaten our health and well-being. My goal in presenting this information is to help you understand the reality of the situation. With this intent you, the reader, must consider the possibility that the writer may be right. If so, then I have done my part.

The media has bombarded us all for so long with half informed information and alleged facts concerning ozone that it is hard to begin to comprehend the true story.

The much-maligned ozone locked in smog is nothing but bad. However, down-to-earth scientific research points in an altogether different direction. The utterances from the medical community, the government and the media never change. Once that sinks in, you may be more receptive to realizing how short-changed and victimized we have all been. This book strives to clarify controversy and preposterous misconceptions and attitudes toward Nature's precious gift to us, Ozone.

We have been had by the society we live in because we have been encouraged to believe in a supposed right way that is just plain wrong. We were had by a mudslide of propaganda by a media that pounces on and promotes anything that can be looked upon as bad rather than looking at something in more than one way. It all depends on how something is presented to us. Negative information is negative information. It sits in our mind as a bad thing because we have heard it over and over for so long that we no longer question the accuracy of the information.

Ask yourself this question: Is what I am presenting in this book to good to be true? Not at all. It is simply going further into the subject of ozone and discovering positive information. Moreover, it is demonstrated repeatedly and scientifically unimpeachable. That is the revelation within these pages. Revelation, in the connotation of this work, means to make known truths that were always there in the first place. If the facts I have presented here are finally accepted as truths by some of the scientific community, and at the same time are not suspect by many people, then indeed this book will be an act of revelation.

For those who choose to be the naysayers and doubters about the factual qualities of ozone let them live in a sick home until they come to their senses. I, for one, do not know of another example within the scientific field where there exists such a vast discrepancy between what actually takes place and what is said to take place.
HOW?

Achieving a safer environment, creating healthier surroundings, reducing unneeded and unpleasant consequences in our lives is literally as available to each of us as is the air we breathe. If you remember anything you learned about the air we breathe, you will recall that every time a breath is taken it is not pure oxygen being inhaled. If you have forgotten your science, it is a mixture of gases, some of which might surprise you. The air we breathe is made up of nitrogen (78.09%), oxygen (20.95%) and carbon dioxide (0.03%). In addition, there are trace gases that account for the other 0.93%. These include neon, helium, methane, krypton, hydrogen, xenon and ozone.

From sea level to 18,000 feet, this mixture is fairly uniform. In this region of the atmosphere is where 50% of all these gases are found with the densest being at sea level, measuring 1000 millibars. The mixture begins to become less dense as it ascends. At 18,000 feet it is half as dense as it is at sea level. At 18,000 feet it takes 2 breaths to equal 1 breath at sea level. For example, the elevation of Denver, Colorado is approximately 5,000 feet and therefore has a 20% reduction in density. You must take 5 breaths to equal 4 breaths at sea level. Ascend another 18,000 feet to 36,000 feet and you are now at the top of the troposphere; above you is the stratosphere. It still has air but in ever decreasing amounts.

At the top of the troposphere and for eight miles into the stratosphere is where the action is. This is where we encounter ozone. This is where regular oxygen molecules known as O_2 (2 atoms of oxygen) make up one molecule. This is the same oxygen we need to stay alive. Here ultraviolet light or radiation from the sun bombards these O_2 molecules. When ultraviolet radiation hits O_2, it breaks the bond into two single or separate atoms. These single atoms seek other 2 atom oxygen molecules to form the three atom molecules we call Ozone.

In this process, heat is released and the ozone molecules also absorbing incoming radiation, re-radiating all of this heat back into the stratosphere thus creating a stable stratosphere. However, more important to the inhabitants of our planet, both animal and plant life, is the deflection of and the absorption of ultraviolet radiation. At 36,000 to 75,000 feet ozone saves this planet from the deadly side of sunshine.

Much has been made of the expanding areas of the outer troposphere where ozone has been reduced or has actually disappeared. If this is a natural phenomenon that has occurred before, mass extinction of life on earth is one possibility. The other is the result of the pollution we have been creating at an ever-increasing rate since the early 1800's. If the former is the case, there is little to be done. If the latter is the real cause, we may be able to slow the process allowing nature to rebuild the ozone layer. But it may be too late for that to occur. Only time will tell.

At 36,000 to 75,000 feet, how does pollution create havoc in the ozone layer (also known as the ozonosphere)? The process is really very simple. First of all, about 2 billion years ago plants began to produce abundant free oxygen as a waste gas. This formed a thin layer of ozone close to the surface of the earth. About one billion years ago the formation of a thicker protective ozone layer is what probably allowed plants then animals to move from the oceans to the land.

CFC's or chlorofluoro-carbons, as well as such natural phenomena as volcanic eruptions have an effect on the ozone layer. Volcanic activity throws sulfuric acid high into the atmosphere where it enhances the destructiveness of the chlorine chemicals. It is this activity that does the real damage to the ozonosphere.

When CFC's are released into the atmosphere then rise up into the stratosphere (36,000 to 75,000 feet), the ultraviolet radiation is intense enough to split the CFC molecule that results in the freeing of chlorine atoms. The chlorine then attacks an ozone molecule (O_3) stealing one-oxygen atom to form chlorine monoxide. The former ozone molecule (O_3) is less one atom and is a simple O_2 molecule. In the meantime, the chlorine monoxide molecule finds a free oxygen atom. In the collision of the two, the one oxygen atom leaves the chlorine and joins the free oxygen atom resulting in another ordinary oxygen molecule of O_2. The chlorine atom is now free to steal another oxygen atom from another ozone molecule, and so on.

The mathematics are fairly simple: one chlorine atom destroys one ozone molecule leaving behind an ordinary oxygen molecule, O_2. Then instead of the ozone molecule being reconstituted with a free oxygen atom joining the ordinary O_2 molecule, the free oxygen atom joins the oxygen atom stolen by the chlorine and results in another ordinary oxygen molecule. We have just lost one molecule of ozone.

Without the chlorine atom present, we would have had one ozone molecule and one free oxygen atom capable of joining an ordinary O_2 to form ozone in the presence of ultraviolet radiation, thus yielding two ozone molecules. The chlorine leaves behind 2 ordinary O_2-oxygen molecules. In essence, our outer defense zone of ozone is reduced in its ability to protect life on earth from ultraviolet radiation.

So far we know that oxygen and ultraviolet radiation create a molecule called ozone, a form of oxygen that serves to shield the earth. However, there is a second form of ozone. It is composed of 3 oxygen atoms. It is not well loved mainly because of its origins. It is properly described as *low-level ozone* or *surface ozone.*

This is the bad ozone. The ozone talked about and recorded in air quality reports. What makes this ozone different? *Low level* or *surface ozone* is formed when volatile organic compounds (oxygen and nitrogen oxides) chemically react in the presence of sunlight and warmth. Note that sunlight is involved but not ultraviolet radiation. This *low level* or *surface ozone* has its sources from motor vehicle and power plant emissions, landfills and solvents. CFC's are used as coolants in air conditioners and refrigeration systems. They are also used in cleaning solvents. This ozone will never have that after-a-summer-storm aroma that characterizes the type of ozone found out there in the rarified ozonosphere simply because it is made from different ingredients and by an entirely different process. This smelly, obnoxious, unhealthy surface ozone has 3 atoms of oxygen.

Molecules that contain 3 atoms of oxygen are labeled with the name of ozone. Consequently, good ozone gets a bad rap and ends up being a scapegoat. Here we have the major misunderstanding of ozone, and it's all in the name.

The third form of ozone is the type formed when lightning strikes the earth.

So, ozone has three distinctly different sources that can produce it. However, the most natural method is the one based on the action of ultraviolet light and oxygen. This method does not produce any harmful or potentially harmful byproducts.

H_20, or water, has a similar name problem. Think about it. Pour a glass of water from a bottle labeled as *distilled*, one from a mountain spring, and finally one from a polluted swamp near some industrial site. All three glasses are filled with water. Although each contains H_20, or water, they are significantly different in many aspects.

So it is with ozone. Each from a different source, all are 0_3, all are ozone, but each is unique. In hearing discussions about ozone remember water especially the spring water. Then remember that there is a natural process for producing ozone. So why not try to produce ozone as naturally as possible?

Why would anyone concern themselves with ozone and its production? This is probably a good question if you are not familiar with the knowledge and science around which this book is written. However, because the health and welfare of your family and you are of paramount importance, and you certainly are concerned about their nutrition and their future, then ozone should be of great interest to you.

Ozone is a more powerful oxidizing agent than oxygen. In the presence of water or water vapor it is a powerful bleaching agent. Ozone acts more rapidly than hydrogen peroxide, chlorine or sulfur dioxide and ozone is active at very low temperatures. It is 5,000 times faster than chlorine in its ability to provide bacterial and viral disinfecting. Using the natural approach to production of ozone actually results in safer, far more flexible applications and far more economical costs for users. Finally, ozone is coming of age!

CHAPTER 9

OZONE AS A DEFENDER OF YOUR HOME AND YOUR FAMILY'S HEALTH

Ozone is not a cure-all. All ozone can do is eliminate the cause of a sick home whether it is a moldy room, a mildewy closet, or a fungi-ridden house. Ozone can kill dust mites and destroy their problem causing feces. Ozone can eliminate the source of most foul and noxious odors such as animal urine and feces. Ozone can rid a new or remodeled home of toxic degassing chemicals created by the very materials that are used in new construction and remodeling.

How does ozone actually do these tasks? In technical terms the process is known as *oxidation* and ozone is known as an *oxidizer*. It is a more powerful oxidizer that ordinary oxygen, O_2. Oxidation is a process in which oxygen is caused to combine with other molecules. The oxygen used may be as elemental oxygen (O_2 or O_3.) Most oxidation occurs with the release of energy such as igniting wood or petroleum. Other forms of oxidation include corrosion, decay and respiration. The oxidation of organic compounds with a form of oxygen, particularly ozone, appear to proceed through free radical chain reactions that are very complex and are not completely understood.

What constitutes an organic compound? Everything that is carbon based is an organic compound with the exception of some simple carbon compounds such as carbon dioxide. Carbon dioxide is usually treated as an inorganic compound. Nearly everything derived from petroleum, wood, plants or produced in a laboratory as well as all living organisms from bacteria, viruses, molds, and dust mites, urines, feces and just about every foul odor or germ that is carbon based. Caulking, glues, wallpaper, paints, insulation and various gases produced by them, the urea products used for wafer board, strand board, plywood board, carpeting, pads, and drapes are all carbon based. All are potential breeding grounds for other carbon based life forms.

Foodstuffs are all carbon based as well as the pesticides and microbes, such as E-Coli, plus all the chemicals that have been used on these foods from the farm to the market to the dinner table. Meat, chicken and fish are all carbon based. The odors of rancidity and decay are also carbon based resulting from exposure to oxygen, O_2. Spores, germs and other detrimental life forms are of the same carbon basis and are imbedded in your clothing. They are accumulated from wherever you have been.

To remove, eradicate, deodorize or sanitize all these items, from the house, the table, and the wardrobe, you will need something that will kill the viruses, bacteria, other toxins and eliminate or neutralize phenol, pesticides and all foul odors. It is the oxidizing effect of naturally generated ozone that can do just this and do it better and with much greater safety than any form of household disinfectant or chlorine. It does its job without leaving harmful residues or chemicals.

We know that ozone has 3 atoms of oxygen comprising the molecule. When this super-charged form of oxygen is unleashed it literally wants to find carbon based gases and solids. After all, ozone is quite unstable having 3 atoms. It wants to become a stable 2-atom molecule. When ozone finds a carbon-based problem molecule, it destroys it with great efficiency. Ozone simply oxidizes the complex carbon based molecules. From the degassing of new construction and remodeling, to molds, mildew, viruses, feces, urines, dust mites, germs and foul odors, Ozone does its job and when completed, reverts to oxygen, O_2.

This process repeats itself until the job is done. They find formaldehyde degassing from your paneling and away goes that 3rd atom to wreak its havoc in our behalf. Over in the corner mildew is emitting its musty odor while enjoying a little humidity and some oxygen. But ozone has homed in on it. Again, devastation as the O_3 sheds an atom as it attacks the very structure of the mildew. This search and destroy mission continues as long as these unstable O_3 ozone molecules are released.

In the clothes closet, they will attack the smelly shoe odors, the odors of perspiration and body odors. In the bathroom, they are creating havoc on molds, mildew and little critters only seen under a microscope. Throughout the house this battle will be fought. All those little ozones will be happy 2-atom molecules of oxygen and those 3rd atoms will have done their job, then re-group with other loners and become stable two atom oxygen molecules again.

OZONE SAFE AND HEALTHFUL USE

Occasionally there arise various claims about the healthfulness of just about everything on this earth. Every time such claims or questions surface it would appear that we are all doomed or saved, depending on our response. There are those who claim that ingesting this vitamin or that mineral will do this or that for health, sexuality or longevity. Whether it is vegetarianism or herbalism, all of these various selections have, in the long run, proven one thing over and over. If something works for one person, it may or may not work for the next person. Too much oxygen is bad for you. It can kill you. Too much water can be bad for you. There are those who may react adversely to what is another's favorite food.

Over the years there have been those who believe ozone is a miracle form of oxygen and that breathing it constantly is the path to health. *WE DO NOT RECOMMEND EXCEEDING THE PUBLISHED SAFETY LEVELS.* Through the process of oxidation, we know that ozone will reduce and eliminate fungus, molds, bacteria, viruses and will neutralize toxic gases coming from the numerous synthetic materials that are found in older and newer homes.

To achieve positive results from ozone (and not over-do a good and useful tool) we only consider ozone produced in the same manner as an unpolluted earth produced it to protect life on earth long before Nature had do deal with today's pollutions and poisons we bring into our homes, put in the air, dump on the earth and pour into our lakes, streams, rivers, oceans and every aquifer known.

In Nature's own inimitable way, we have been given a weapon to use to correct our ill-advised and shortsighted human ways. This is the reason we produce ozone using a proprietary method of ultraviolet ray production and oxygen. This method may not produce enormous quantities of ozone, but it also does not produce potentially dangerous and lethal by-products produced by the corona discharge and plasma methods. This natural production from ultraviolet rays and oxygen results in safe and useful levels of ozone without residues and side effects to worry about.

What are safe levels to use to achieve good, effective results? Again, let us look to Nature for some guidance. In rural, unpolluted, unpopulated areas the normal concentration of ozone is .01-.03 parts per million parts of air. In cities without smog, the amount drops to 0.1 ppm. However, if we are in a city with smog, the ozone level will rise to .05 ppm or more for short periods of time. However, this ozone is produced as a result of warm air, sunlight, and the emissions from autos, power plants, factories and solvents to name just a few of the culprits.

Yes, it is ozone but the similarity is much like that between distilled water (pure H_2O) and a glass of water from a drainage ditch in an industrial area. Both are H_2O, but there is a huge difference between the two. Of the sources of ozone production available, only one is a safe, natural source and excels far beyond all others. That method is the proprietary SCO Technologies Medallion Healthy Home method.

The U.S. Occupational Safety and Health Administration believe workers can be exposed to .01 ppm per 8-hour day of ozone. The Environmental Protection Agency (EPA) has set the ozone exposure level at .12 ppm per 1-hour, per day, or .08 ppm per 8 hours, and the Canadian Standards Association (CSA) has set .04 ppm as the limit for household ozone levels. The American Society of Heating, Refrigeration and Air Conditioning Engineers (ASHRAE) recommend a maximum of .05 ppm. In the highlands of New Mexico, 0.05 to 0.08-ppm ozone levels are common as a result of the intense high altitude sunlight catalysis of hydrocarbons of pine trees. For centuries people in this area have boasted of their great longevity.

These concentrations of ozone may be called *safe concentrations*. However, scientific studies demonstrate that for effective decontamination of the air, and to prevent the survival and regeneration of biological organisms in the contaminated area, levels of .5 to .8 ppm must be achieved. However, no humans, pets or plants can be present. Thus, these studies do support the use of ozone, but only when used in a safe and controlled application. Again, it is only with the methods and technologies developed by SCO Technologies and the Medallion Healthy Home System that a truly effective and safe use of ozone can result in a Healthy Home.

The studies supporting these facts include;

Dyas, A.; Boughton, B.J.; Das, B.C. 1983, Ozone Killing Action Against Bacterial and Fungal Species; Microbiological Testing of a Domestic Ozone Generator. *Journal of Clinical Pathology*. 36:1102-1104.

Foarde, K.; van Osdell, D.; and Steiber, R. 1997. Investigation of Gas-Phase Ozone as a Potential Biocide. *Applied Occupational Environmental Hygiene.* 12(8): 535-542.

• Some data suggest that low levels of ozone may reduce airborne concentrations and inhibit the growth of some biological organisms while ozone is present, but ozone concentrations would have to be 5—10 times higher than public health standards allow before the ozone could decontaminate the air sufficiently to prevent survival and regeneration of the organisms once the ozone is removed (Dyas, et al., 1983; Foarde, et al.; 1997.)

• Even at high concentrations, ozone may have no effect on biological contaminants embedded in porous material such as duct lining or ceiling tiles (Foarde et al, 1997.) In other words, ozone produced by ozone generators may inhibit the growth of some biological agents while it is present, but it is unlikely to fully decontaminate the air unless concentrations are high enough to be a health concern if people are present. Even with high levels of ozone, contaminants embedded in porous material may not be affected at all.

These studies present proof positive that ozone is effective as a biocide and will create a healthier home. It also makes it very clear that to achieve effectiveness, it must be introduced into the home by trained technicians using a system consisting of equipment that will do the job. This is why SCO Technologies does not allow the general public to buy and use their specialized and proprietary equipment. Only technicians trained by SCO Technologies Medallion Healthy Homes are qualified to do so.

Safety is our utmost concern. That includes you, your family, your pets and even your houseplants. Do not be misled by anyone or any company claiming that ozone generators will or can do this or that. To properly do the job, we must exceed safe levels in order to achieve our treatment goals. Only the SCO Technologies Medallion Healthy Homes System can do what must be done in a safe and timely fashion.

This is not a do-it-yourself technology. Don't waste your money or such efforts. Do it right—do it safely, and enjoy a healthier home with your family, your pets and even your houseplants!

THE SICK HOME SYNDROME

To designate a home as a *sick home* is not an exact science, and therefore is a very complex undertaking. Only the findings of information assembled by the owner/occupant and possibly their doctor can make that determination.

THE CRITERIA

Sensitive reactions, though not fully understood, may be the effect of numerous irritants resulting in severe emotional distress and serious chronic illness.

There are many different things in the average home that can contribute to the *sick home syndrome* such as odors, allergy causing molds, fungus, degassing materials, animal urine, feces and dander, dust mites, life threatening bacteria(s) and viruses. Separately, or worse yet, mixed combinations of contaminates that can number in the thousands. Subsequently, it is usually impossible to isolate and deal with any one of the numerous potential sources of the problem(s).

THE ANSWER

SCO Medallion Healthy Home's solution is to employ a high saturation blanket treatment to address the wide spectrum of potential contaminates that is causing the *sick home syndrome*. The SCO Medallion Healthy Home proprietary pure (clean) ozone treatment system is the only known method capable of dealing with, eliminating and destroying the broad spectrum of carbon-based elements that are the cause of the *sick home syndrome*.

OUR PRIMARY GOAL

Is to cure the *sick home syndrome* to the best of our professional ability. Our pledge to you is to conduct our business with the highest degree of consideration at all times; to carry out each home application with the same concern and professionalism, as we would demand to be carried out in our own homes.

In many cases, our experience has shown that after treatment the problem(s) in the *sick home* has been cured, however the isolation of the specific contaminate(s) was not identified. Nevertheless, our results were positive.

Although our success rate is approximately 96%, from time to time we encounter problem homes with complex contamination that just cannot be isolated and therefore, is beyond our capabilities at this time.

Human and animal urine is the perfect example of a very common offensive compound that creates problems.

In 1500 cubic centimeters or urine, the average daily excretion of the normal human adult male, there are 60 grams of dissolved substances, including 30 grams of urea, which is residue from the body; 15 grams of sodium chloride and lesser quantities of potassium, sulfuric acid, phosphoric acid, ammonia and other substances.

In animals, the overall amount is less in volume. However, animal urine is more highly concentrated. Every time a cat or dog urinates it leaves behind a thimble full of a very highly concentrated potent smelling residue that bonds to the fabric in rugs, upholstery and drapes in the form of *carbon molecules.*

Carbon molecules are food (so-to-speak) for the Super Charged Oxygen System. The system generates O_3, which, with the help of the Super Charged Oxygen System's specifically compounded oxidizing solution, seeks out the offending molecules and oxidizes and destroys them on the spot.

Basically, all offensive odors have one main ingredient in common, carbon molecules. Therefore, the Super Charged Oxygen System is *lethal* when it comes to destroying offensive odors.

HOW THE SYSTEM WORKS IN DEALING WITH OFFENSIVE ODORS IN THE ENVIRONMENT

The system works best in ambient temperatures of 65—85 degrees. Locate and isolate the primary area of the offending odor. If an extreme case, use the Super Charged Oxygen System Oxidizing Solution, in a very gentle mist, to cover the odorous area to be treated.

The Oxidizing Solution is a specifically formulated, environmentally safe, molecular compound designed to be attracted to the receptor site and bond with carbon and other odor causing molecules in rugs, drapes, upholstered furniture plus other surfaces and materials. It is the Oxidizing Solution that lays out the pathway of destruction directly to the offending odor molecule(s). Super Charged Oxygen now has a fast lane to the culprit causing it to disintegrate into ashes by the process of oxidation.

By using Super Charged Oxygen oxidation and atomization there is no cover up with perfume-like air fresheners. These air fresheners are, in themselves, another form of odor. In fact, as they dissipate they can compound the problem. Therefore, using air fresheners alone will not do the job because air fresheners dissipate in a short time leaving the offending odor intact.

The Super Charged Oxygen System loves to oxidize and destroy these offending problems and odors:

Smoke, Fungus, Mold, Viruses, Urine, Pollen, Bacteria, Hydrocarbons, Mildew, Spores, Dust mites and their feces, Yeasts and most chemical manufacturing residue odors in new rugs, paints and paneling, such as formaldehyde and all those previously mentioned elsewhere.

CHAPTER 10

THE EPILOGUE

The research and experiments with ozone came quite by accident. One could call it serendipity. In 1985, in the process of the development of the Ultra 3000 Photo Plate system, a polymer-curing device that resulted in the ability to cure polymer resins in 20 seconds rather than 10 minutes (this was a major breakthrough,) we discovered the production of ozone as a byproduct. This discovery led us to the realization that ozone has practical value in brand new applications. We were familiar with it as a superior method of purifying water, but further research opened up new and far more exciting and really useful applications. As our interest in ozone increased, we became involved in its ability to deal with odor control by eliminating (destroying) the very source causing the odors that is necessary to the breeding bacteria and viruses within molds, and so on. It became viable to produce ozone equipment.

The highest concentration of ozone production (and the costliest) was to use the corona discharge method that we proceeded to use in our production equipment, just as everyone else was using, until a major catastrophe happened to me.

One of our customers returned a machine for rebuilding/maintenance. I wanted to service this machine to examine the unit thoroughly because the unit had had hard service. In the process of changing out the generators, I noticed a large amount of wet residue of a brown-yellow nature that had accumulated in the bottom of the unit. I proceeded to remove the generators for replacement. As I reached under the generator to unfasten the connection, I submerged the back of my hand in that yellow-brown accumulation in the bottom of the unit.

The shocking, excruciating pain I felt was indescribable. I yanked my hand out and ran to a water faucet about 20 feet away. I turned the water on full force to wash away the residue. After a while I removed my hand from under the faucet and looked at the damage, not knowing what I would find. The pain had subsided to some extent. However, it was still nearly unbearable. I looked at the top of my hand and where I had normal pink skin, the top of my hand was now yellow-brown. I quickly split an aloe Vera leaf and applied a coating over the surface of my hand. All this time my mind was racing; "what in damnation did I just get into?" Then it hit me. I had covered my hand with a huge amount of concentrated nitric acid! The yellow-brown gunk was the result (byproduct) of the manufacturing process of the corona discharge method of manufacturing ozone.

In order to confirm my suspicions, I scraped up some of the residue, mixed it with water and dropped a piece of copper wire into the solution. There it was! Just as I had suspected, that yellow-brown vapor coming out of the solution was an indication of nitric acid. That was the moment a crucial final decision was made. Our company would never participate, in any manner whatsoever, in the manufacturing of corona discharge ozone generators or any other ozone generators that had the ability to generate these dangerous by-products. I knew what I had just experienced was not going to ever happen to anyone else if I could help it.

We recalled every corona discharge unit we had every manufactured with the understanding that they would be replaced when our new SCO Technologies Proprietary UV pure ozone generators became operational.

It was now time to diligently move forward and pursue our goal of producing the best and most sophisticated pure ozone producing equipment in the world. This type of equipment simply did not exist. However, in the development of the Ultra 3000 system, we had accumulated a huge amount of information and knowledge about ozone and the production of ozone.

We put this knowledge to work. Our goal was simply, "if we are going to do it, we are going to do it right or not do it at all." Our commitment was straightforward—we have to do it better than has ever been done before, not just with financial gain in mind, but a product that is also a huge benefit to mankind.

Our ultimate goal was to produce ozone as residue-free as possible and without dangerous or hazardous gasses. This is keeping in line with the ACGIH (American Conference of Governmental Industrial Hygienists) whose standards are more stringent than OSHA (Occupational Safety and Health Administration.)

On-going research and development had brought about many innovations. The housing (cabinet) that contains the ozone generators and affiliated parts and materials are of the best surgical stainless steel with a very specific finish enhancing the quality of ozone production. By using MSA (Mine Safety Appliances, established in 1914) equipment for testing, differentiating detections could be tabulated and recorded. Since most commercial testing laboratories do not have the full capabilities to test for ozone and ozone production concerning related residues, we felt more comfortable with our own MSA test findings.

The lamps (generators) are of a specialized composition of fused quartz lamp tubes to maximize performance, to withstand the rigors of expansion and contraction, and to produce specific wavelengths without cancellation. Specifically designed and constructed trouble-free ballasts to drive the generators are used.

In summary, it took 2 years of research and development to bring, what to my knowledge, is the purest, most uncontaminating ozone production equipment in the world into reality.

I stand by all of the above. Unless it has the Medallion name on it, it is not producing the most pure and uncontaminated ozone possible. Only Medallion ozone production systems are designed and engineered to assure you of such pure, natural ozone production.

THE COMPANY
SCO TECHNOLOGIES MEDALLION
HEALTHY HOMES LTD

The author would be remiss if he were to omit the business opportunity available to an aspiring entrepreneur; the opportunity to do and be everything he or she wants to be. The opportunity simply does not get any better; it's the best of both worlds.

Building a business of your own with the Medallion Healthy Home system gives an ambitious person the opportunity to participate in making people's lives better and, in the process, you also have the opportunity to become financially independent.

Presently, the Company is allocating Exclusive Territories throughout the United States and Canada to those who are farsighted and have the ambition to become recognized business people and leaders in their community. The demographics for the allocations are as follows:

FRANCHISE DEALER TERRITORY:
Franchised Dealer Territories are areas that have an approximate 125,000 population and approximately 50,000 households. These territories can be increased proportionately if the dealer desires. An area this size will encompass a thriving community with potential business everywhere from sick homes, sick buildings, schools, automobiles, motor homes, boats and anywhere and everywhere there are nasty odors, molds, mildew

and toxic viruses and bacteria have become a problem and threat to health.

Currently, the Franchised Dealer Territory is unlimited. However, in a very short period of time the areas are going to become limited. Dealers may expand their areas within a region if, in fact, additional territories are available.

REGIONAL MASTER FRANCHISE

The Regional Master Franchise encompasses an area that may consist of between 4,000,000 and 15,000,000 people and has the opportunity to establish a number of Franchised Dealer Territories within his Region to his benefit. Also the Regional Master Franchise has the opportunity to receive a fee for establishing the Franchise Dealer as well as receiving an on-going royalty from their business. This can be very rewarding.

The management of Medallion Healthy Homes Ltd and the author feel that the time has come for the public to address the danger and horrors of the home environment because we now have the proper tools available, at a reasonable cost. The new technology developed by Medallion Healthy Homes Ltd is of the utmost benefit to mankind. This opportunity also enables the entrepreneur with the "want-to" and "stick-to-it-ness" the most beneficial rewards by becoming an active player in this new field.

For more information on how to be a part of the Medallion Healthy Homes Ltd family of franchises, please contact 425-672-4808.

THE EXPERIENCE OF OTHERS

I have never been a big fan of testimonials. However, these are a little different. These individuals have been adamant in asking me to include their experiences, and since many were involved in letting me perfect the SCO Technology in their homes, I feel I owe it to them, along with my sincere thanks and appreciation.

September 6, 1998

I am writing to thank you for the recent "de-odorizing" services you provided to my clients and myself. I am the first to admit that when I saw the flyer regarding "Super Charged Oxygen" I was quite skeptical. I tend to think most claims of wondrous success are overstated. YOURS WERE NOT!

I have encountered many homes over the years suffering from strong pet odors; this listing of mine in Kirkland however, was among the worst. It clearly had nearly overpowering pet dander and urine odor. In the past, the property would have had to be priced substantially lower to adjust for it, or replace the carpeting.

With little to lose and lots to gain we decided to try it. The results were quite amazing! This split level home had a concrete slab basement floor under the carpet and standard wood subflooring upstairs. The odor was GONE from the upstairs and SUBSTANTIALLY removed from the lower level. I suspect the only reason it lingered there was that the smell had permeated the concrete.

The property sold soon after we had the "Super Charged Oxygen" treatment, and I credit it in large part to your services. I will call you again on my next "stinky" listing.

Thanks again.

Yours truly,
Ekik Noyd
Coldwell Banker Bain Associates

November 12, 1998

I am writing to thank you for all that you and your line of Super Charged Oxygen machines have done for both my wife and me. Our business has almost doubled in the past 1½ years without doubling our labor. Keeping our 6 machines working constantly has been very rewarding.

After the first of the year, we will be ordering 2 more ozonator machines from you and I am happy to say that we will not need to finance these, as we will be paying cash. We are particularly interested in the newer models you have discussed with us.

Thanks for everything!

Sincerely,
Kevin and Shanai Cole, Owners
Enviro-Tech, Inc.

March, 1999

This short note is just to let you know how much my wife and I appreciated your SCO equipment.

My wife has been suffering from allergy-like symptoms for a long time; terrible headaches, sneezing, coughing, runny nose. We thought these might be from the mold in our house or the carpeting.

After using the Super Charged Oxygen System in our house for a couple of hours, then airing out for a few minutes, there was a noticeable smell of freshness in the house. We used it again after a month and my wife is now feeling a lot better.

No more headaches, coughing or sneezing. Her symptoms have disappeared! She says she now feels she's a better person. Our thanks to you! We strongly believe every home should have one of these Super Charged Oxygen Systems.

Sincerely,
Sully and Karen Sullivan

March, 1999

I would like to inform you of the service and performance of your Super Charged Oxygen machines.

When everything else we tried failed, we used them on diesel and gasoline fueled boats and they performed exceptionally well. The diesel-fueled boat had been in storage for 2 years. Your machine took all the diesel smell and mold from the interior of the boat and left a clean smell throughout the interior and engine room of the boat.

The gasoline-fueled boat didn't smell as bad, but had an exhaust/engine smell throughout the inside, which we had not been able to remove until we used your Super Charged Oxygen machine.

Again, we thank you and highly recommend your equipment to any boat owner who has encountered the same problems we have.

Thank you again.

Sincerely,
Gerald T. Dishneau Sr., President
FLEET CARE, INC.

November, 1999

I am writing this letter to give testimonial to the effectiveness of Medallion Healthy Homes system in eliminating strong and persistent cooking odors. The cooking odor I'm referring to was the result of a "mistake" I made when cooking a lamb roast one afternoon. I put the roast in the oven and then headed back to our office (which is only a few minutes from the house) to complete a couple of tasks. These tasks should have taken only 20-30 minutes, but I ended up doing other things and forgetting about the roast. When I did get home 4 hours later, I knew as soon as I drove into the garage that I was in trouble. I opened the garage door and found the house completely filled with a brown, oily smelling smoke.

We have a fairly big house, about 5,000 sq. ft., and every room including those in the finished basement, was filled with this oily smelling smoke. I immediately opened all doors and windows and was eventually able to somewhat clear the smoke; but the smell wouldn't go away. I tried several different aerosol sprays and even a small air purifier that I had. Nothing worked! We went to bed that night with that smell and woke up again the morning with that smell. Even our clothes reeked! It was awful. After two days of living like this, I had had enough. I called a friend of mine to see if he had any ideas of how to kill the stench and he told me about Medallion. I called them and they came out the next day.

They arrived just as I was leaving for the office in the morning. I don't know exactly what they did but when I came home that night the house smelled great! That horrible oily smell was gone from every room. Even my clothes smelled good. The whole house had a fresh smell, which the Medallion people explained was a very low concentration of residual ozone such as you might get after a thunderstorm. I found it quite pleasant.

Medallion, I can't thank you enough!

Yours truly,
Ms. Deborah Abossein
Bellevue, WA

January, 2000

My wife, Jane, and I wish to express our sincere appreciation for the wonderful ozone-producing product that your company manufacturers. On two occasions we used your OZONATOR to remove unpleasant odors, both times with complete success.

The first time, our dogs had cornered a skunk under our new modular home. Needless to say, "the odor was *OVERPOWERING*"—both in the home and on the dogs. We operated your OZONATOR in our home for 24 hours, and much to our surprise and delight, the smell was eliminated completely! In fact, the modular home smelled fresh, like the air after a thunderstorm. It was truly an "act of God" or maybe it was due to "an active dog."

The second time, we used the OZONATOR to eliminate a strong "dog-odor" in our log home. While the home was under construction, before doors were installed, our dogs used a favorite corner for sleeping, and for entertaining guests, some of whom we suspect were not housebroken. Over a period of time, a strong, ever-present odor built up. Your OZONA-TOR cured the problem in short order.

Thank you again for producing such an effective, easy to use product; and for helping to transform both of our homes into enjoyable living spaces.

Sincerely,
Ken Holmes & Jane Rosewood

HEALTHY HOME CHECKLIST:

LIVING ROOM:

Carpet
Entry way mat
All hardwood surfaces
Between and under couch and chair cushions
Around picture window
Curtains and blinds

KITCHEN:

On top and underneath all appliances
The sink and underneath the sink
Tops of cabinets and shelves inside

Countertop surfaces
Linoleum and hardwood floors
Dirty dishes
Inside refrigerator
Compactor
Garbage cans
Waste baskets

FAMILY ROOM:

Same as living room

BEDROOMS:

Under the bed
All bedding
Carpet
Dresser and table surfaces
Around the window
Curtains and blinds
Inside closets

BATHROOMS:

Around tub/shower
Toilet and base of toilet
Tile, linoleum, or carpet flooring
Countertops
Sink and under sink
Cabinets and drawers
Closets
Wastebaskets

HALLWAYS:

Carpet
Linen/coat closet

ABOUT THE AUTHOR

The author would like to introduce himself to you. The following is a brief and up-to- date synopsis.

Daniel Molleker, Chairman of SCO Technologies Medallion Healthy Homes Ltd

1933—Born and raised on a grain, dairy and livestock farm in Kansas where it was necessary to acquire the mechanical skills related to maintaining machinery in good repair and working condition and improvising when necessary, or as needed. This practical and applied experience and knowledge became the foundation of a long and successful career.

1950-1960—Began my working career in the oil and gas service industry oil field construction, and sales, and progressed to management. Also obtained a pilot license, owning and operating single and multi-engine aircraft, and have over 5,000 hours flying experience as pilot in command.

1961-1966—Formed Molleker Service Company, an oil field service company servicing the oil and gas industry. Designed and developed the adjustable under pressure automatic weir siphon to maintain consistent water levels in pressurized oil and water separation vessels. Also designed and developed the Molleker Company cathodic protection system to arrest corrosion in tank, pipeline and casing installations.

The company was sold at a considerable profit in 1966. Remained actively involved in the exploration, development and production in the oil and gas industry to this date.

1967—Designed and developed the REDI-EDDY and ULTRA POWER devices. These devices were engineered to allow the operation of 110-volt power tools, fast battery charges and welders from any car or pickup alternator by bypassing the regulator. The Ultra Power Company was sold at a profit in 1973.

1972—Designed and developed a rotary cinerating furnace for roasting precious metal concentrates and a centrifugal force caustic liquid, silver recovery system for Superior Precious Metals Refinery while being instrumental in arranging financing for operations, expansion and dealing in precious metals. This company was sold to an international refining group in 1982.

1972-1984—Expanded my interest in the coin-collecting field by purchasing Firdale Coin and Stamp in Edmonds, Washington as a dealer of numismatic, philatelic, precious metals, jewelry and gemstones. Created commemorative medallions of the Alaska pipeline in gold and also confirmation medallions of Latvia and the Pathways of Jesus. A recognized numismatic appraiser and a National Associated Fellow of the Smithsonian Institution.

1983—Developed story boards for the first voice speaking interacting children's computer learning programs utilizing the Commodore Pet, Vic 20 #64, Amiga 500 and the Amiga 2000 systems for CPSI, a computer software company specializing in L-P, Little People programs. This company was merged with Decker Resources Ltd., a publicly trading company, in 1986. Instrumental in orchestrating the merger and arranging the necessary financing.

1987—Designed and developed a high-speed (10 second) polymer-curing device for Artistic Photo Plate Creations, Inc. This machine is sold worldwide as an instant polymer coating cure in the photo and circuit board industry. As an offshoot of this machine, the SCO-03 ozone generator was perfected.

Designed, developed and patented the Artistic Photo Precision Circle Cutter, a device used in the photo and gasket industry to cut precise close tolerance circles. Arranged the initial Public Offering for Artistic Photo Place Corporation, and the listing of the company on the Vancouver Stock Exchange.

1990-1991—Through on-going involvement in the oil and gas industry, I was instrumental in designing and developing the New Lift-Fluid Transfer System for oil field application. This system moves fluid faster and more economically than conventional pumping systems. The rights to this system technology were sold to Swiss Technique, a public company, at a substantial profit.

1992-Present—Responsible organizer in forming Good Pace, Inc. for the purpose of designing, developing and manufacturing electric vehicles and electric drive systems. Designed and developed the SCAT ABOUT series vehicles, the EAGLE vehicles and the Certified Good Pace Electric Drive Systems.

This system is the only system whereby all components are designed to compliment one another for better performance. The controls are designed to be compatible with the vonMolleker motor and are the only controls of this type with built in internal regeneration. The DC-DC converter is capable of continuous operation with a range of 65—144 V DC input to 13.5 V DC—40 amp output with an operation frequency that does not interfere with radio reception. The charger is a bulk temperature compensated charger with equalizing and maintenance modes to work within the system. The Guardian is exactly that—it guards the entire system against damage by sensing potential damaging overloads.

This company was acquired by a public trading company as a subsidiary. On June 6, 1998, the author along with Mr. Mark Isaak applied for a patent of the integrated fuel cell with static fuel cell and rotating magnets. This patent (#5,923,106) was granted on July 13, 1999. On December 2, 1999 a second patent (#6,005,322) was also granted for an integrated fuel cell electric motor.

At this writing, patent searches have been made and appropriate patent filings and applications are in the process for 1) Methodology Patent for treatment of sick buildings and homes with our proprietary ozone equipment, and 2) the pure ozone generation equipment.

The authors have also written the following books:

The Guardian
Turning Over a New Leaf
The Medallion Solution

In the works:
Patriotic Parasites—a book about Social Security

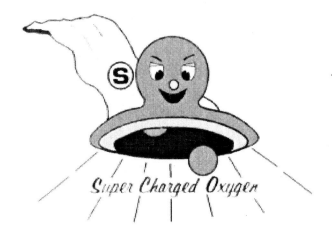

Super Charged Oxygen

Hi!
I'm O.Z.

I'm the new kid on the block

I love to cure sick homes! It's what I was designed for,
and it's what I do best!

Meet me at my website:
www.medallion-healthyhomes.com
Or, call me at 425-672-4808

Let's get acquainted!
See you soon!

O.Z.